# ENEMY FOR A BRAIN

## ZARA BETH

# CONTENTS

# TRIGGER WARNINGS

This book contains scenes describing and talking about mental illness and disability which may be triggering to those of you who have experienced trauma such as hospital stays, seizures, mental illness, or those who may have family members going through difficult times.

Trigger warnings may include:

- Bullying
- Mental health & mental illness
- Talk of suicide
- Seizures & hospital anecdotes

If you find any of these topics distressing or triggering, please read with caution and make sure to check in with yourself along the way; your mental health is the priority!

Any specific chapters containing distressing scenes are listed below, and I've removed graphic details to make this book as accessible as possible whilst still portraying true events. I want to show the reality of my life with health conditions and hopefully educate people on everything I've learned so far.

**Chapter-Specific Triggers:**

- **Chapter 5** - Depression, suicide, mental illness
- **Chapter 7** - Tic attacks
- **Chapter 11** - Covid-19, contamination OCD, mild references to eating disorders
- **Chapter 13** - Tic attacks, injuries & seizures
- **Chapter 15** - Hate comments & suicide
- **Chapter 17** - Medical trauma, hospital scenes, seizures & paralysis
- **Chapter 21** - Medical examinations
- **Chapter 22** - Seizures

*To all the other neurodivergent humans and invisible disability warriors out there, this is for you :)*

*You are worthy. You are incredible. You are never alone.*

# INTRODUCTION

It feels weird writing a book in the first person. Talking about my own experiences. My own life. Over the past four years, I've become increasingly more comfortable talking to a camera and to the millions of people on the other side of the screen, but I've never before shared the true depths of what really goes on in my life and mind day to day.

So, welcome! I'm Zara, mostly known as *Zara Beth* online, and I'm a content creator, writer and disability advocate who shares my journey online. You may be wondering why my story has any impact, why my experiences should be broadcast to the world, or why they're any different to anyone else's... and all I want to say is 'me too'.

I constantly question my ability to help others, assess my content, and compare myself to other role models we see in the media. I question nearly every day whether I'm doing the right thing, whether my posts focus on the right things, whether I'm too much, too little, and so on.

To be truthful, I feel inferior to most people I see online! I suppose we all do from time to time. But I chose to write this book because I have seen the impact of honesty, of sharing your experiences with those who are going through a similar thing; I know how much hearing somebody's story can change your perspective on what you're going through. I've personally experienced the relief felt after realising that you are, in fact, not alone.

So, I want to give this to you. To the people picking this up who may have chronic illnesses, those with disabilities, anybody who is neurodivergent, or anybody who just wants to learn more about life with health struggles, thank you for picking this book up and being open to learning more. The more we talk, the more we can learn.

In this book, I will talk about my life from start to present, sharing my mental health and disability journey, as well as depicting my outlook on life as a child versus how I feel and think now. I'll take you through a bit of my school life, being bullied and how it affected me, experiencing more friendship breakdowns than I can count on both hands, and discussing how my life changed as my brain became "my enemy". I'll also cover being a wheelchair user, my experiences being paralysed from the neck down, and how it feels to have no control over your body due to neurological conditions. I have also included my most recent struggles, sharing how I've found my identity after years of hurt, learning to accept the irreversible and discussing friendship, neurodiversity, advocacy and sexuality.

If I haven't scared you off already, then please read on! This book has been a roller-coaster of emotions, but without sounding *too* cliche, my experiences have completely changed how I think and how I view life. I wouldn't be where I am without them. So, I give you all that I've learnt and all that I've been through in the hopes of bringing you some new knowledge, a new outlook on life, or maybe some of you can relate to this too. Please remember that you are never, ever alone.

# ONE
# MY HEALTH

First things first… some science!

If you know me already, you'll probably know about my conditions and health struggles, but if not, here's an introduction. I'm most commonly recognised for having something called **Tourette's syndrome** (Tourette's or TS for short), a neurological condition which makes my body move involuntarily and makes me say things I can't control.

The most common misconception of Tourette's is that I swear *all* the time, but this isn't true. The uncontrollable movements and sounds are called tics, not to be mistaken with a "tick" which is a type of bug; these are *very* different things!

> "Tics are sudden twitches, movements, or sounds that people do repeatedly. People who have tics cannot stop their body from doing these things."
> - Centre for Disease Control and Prevention

There are two main types of tics, **vocal** and **motor**. A vocal type of tic can be anything from a cough, a grunt, a *meow*, or saying inappropriate words or even sentences. The inappropriate swearing tics are part of something called **coprolalia**.

Coprolalia (*noun*)
   The involuntary and repetitive use of obscene language.


These are complex tics which are often very difficult to suppress. Unfortunately, despite only 10-15% of people with TS (Tourette's syndrome) experiencing coprolalia, I do have this type of tic. And to be quite frank, it's an absolute pain in the backside.

Despite these tics being sometimes amusing and entertaining, they cause daily problems for all the people suffering with Tourette's. One thing I want people to understand is that this isn't the full extent of Tourette's—swearing isn't the only symptom! I will go into more detail about this later in the book, explaining the true reality behind the scenes.

The other type of tic (aside from vocal) is a motor tic—this is a movement. These are most commonly facial twitches and limb jerking, or they can progress to movements as complex as hitting objects or other people, jumping up and down, and even giving the middle finger. It's important to remember that every person has different tics, and no two people have the same experiences of our condition.


I also have a neurological condition called **FND** which stands for **Functional Neurological Disorder**. This is a rarely-heard-of condition I was diagnosed with in 2021 after suffering from undiagnosed symptoms for years. Despite being classed as a "rare" condition, FND is actually one of the most common reasons for neurological referrals in hospitals. It isn't rare, it's just widely under-diagnosed and unheard of.

FND is a highly complex and misunderstood disorder which causes such a wide range of symptoms that I couldn't cover them in a short paragraph. It looks different for most people, but my main struggles are seizures, paralysis, weakness, tremors, dystonia, brain fog and fatigue.

A common co-morbidity to my other conditions is **dysautonomia**, which is an umbrella term for lots of different conditions affecting the autonomic nervous system.

I've suffered from symptoms of orthostatic intolerance since a very young age, but it had never been diagnosed or properly looked into until recently. I've seen my GP (general practitioner or primary healthcare doctor in the UK) many times about my struggles with showering or standing for a long time because this causes painful "rashes" all over my legs along with lots of pre-syncope symptoms like dizziness. After many appointments, doctors suspected Postural Orthostatic Tachycardia Syndrome, but I'm still yet to receive an official diagnosis of my symptoms.

However, I now know my dizziness, raised heart rate and fainting are symptoms of **orthostatic intolerance,** and the "rashes" are actually blood pooling which happens when the heart doesn't pump blood around the body quickly enough.

Orthostatic intolerance (*noun*)
    The development of symptoms while upright or when going from sitting to standing.

Symptoms include light-headedness, palpitations, fatigue, blurred vision, dizziness, exercise intolerance, chest discomfort, cognitive impairment and syncope (fainting). These commonly appear when standing for too long, after having our limbs lower than our hearts for an extended period or when changing posture.

Figuring out that some of my unexplained symptoms stem from dysautonomia has helped me understand why my body struggles, so I can use this information to treat my symptoms, which can prevent further symptoms from happening altogether. Isn't it lovely when things start to make sense and come together!

I suffer from other chronic symptoms, some of which started after a viral infection, but many of these haven't been fully explained even years into my journey. It's very common for people with chronic illnesses to live without diagnoses or explanations for years of their life, due to misunderstandings, gaslighting, lack of healthcare access, and lack of medical research surrounding more complex conditions.

A chronic illness is a long-term health condition that may not have a cure—this includes but is not limited to conditions such as ME/CFS, EDS, Long-Covid, POTS, arthritis, cystic fibrosis, diabetes and more.

Having a chronic illness has changed my perspective on my daily life completely. If I'm being totally honest, I thought it had ruined my entire life for a while... but after years of learning to manage symptoms and having many ups and downs, I finally feel as though I'm ready to share what it has taught me.

Alongside my neurological conditions, I've also struggled with my mental health from quite a young age. Depression and anxiety are words I became overly used to hearing at the ages of twelve and thirteen, but like most people with mental health struggles, my battles started long before I reached out and received any diagnoses.

Tightly linked with anxiety, depression and Tourette's is OCD. My struggles with sensory issues and repetitive, compulsive behaviours started early in my childhood. Only recently have I managed to understand my brain's needs and found methods to make daily functioning slightly more manageable.

Despite having names (diagnoses) for my mental health struggles, I never felt properly *understood*, and my struggles never seemed to quite fit into any bracket. I was anxious, but still strived to do everything everybody around me was doing. I was depressed, but I so badly wanted to fit in, take part and do things which didn't quite add up in my head. I now look back on this and understand that depression showed up mostly as a coping mechanism when feeling like an outsider or during chronic burnout. Even my OCD felt as though it didn't explain *all* of my struggles with sensory sensitivities and social events.

This was... until I learned about autism.

I have more recently been diagnosed as being **autistic**, which presents very differently in young women (and adults) to children, but many people—like younger, undiagnosed me—don't know this until doing further research. The past few years have been incredibly pivotal for me in many ways; one of them has been finding an explanation for my previous mental, social and sensory struggles through my autism diagnosis!

Everything that had seemed "wrong" about me suddenly made sense. I've spent the past two years analysing and going over my whole life in my head, putting together signs and traits of autism I didn't yet understand. Even though being autistic definitely has its negatives (such as the extreme difficulties I face with functioning in day-to-day life, and the social misconceptions around the autistic label), my diagnosis has given me a huge part of my life back.

After first seeing my content or hearing my medical history, many people assume that I'm "collecting diagnoses" or that I "can't possibly have all of those problems", but it is actually very common to have co-morbid conditions when you are disabled (this means, having multiple conditions which are likely to come hand-in-hand). Since receiving my autism diagnosis, I even better understand my mental health history, which I've now realised all links to my autism in some way or another.

Autism helps to explains my earlier mental health struggles.

While different diagnoses can co-occur and are definitely not synonyms for one another, I feel my ASD interacts with (and sometimes even causes) my anxiety, depression and OCD.

I want to point out that this book does not contain my entire life story or my entire medical history. I have kept some details private and have excluded huge segments of my life for the sake of my privacy and to keep the people in my life anonymous. I choose to share some of my diagnoses and medical history because I want to share my story and help other people find communities who understand what they're going through, but this book is by no means all-inclusive of everything I've dealt with in life.

Even when people share a lot online, it's important to remember that we all have battles and hidden struggles which go on behind the scenes. Be kind to those around you, and never assume anything about somebody's life or mindset purely based on what you can physically see.

~

After writing this chapter, I admit this may seem like a lengthy list of labels, especially to those who don't have multiple conditions themselves—but alas, this is how my brain works! Labels aren't necessary if you don't feel that they would personally benefit you, but they're also nothing to be afraid of. Finding a reason for all the ways I've struggled my entire life and having names for the symptoms I suffer with explains why I constantly struggle to function.

Diagnoses give us that much-needed validation that our minds or bodies are indeed different, and that this isn't our fault. My autism diagnosis felt easier to accept than my Tourette's and FND diagnoses because after lots of research, I already *knew* my brain worked in an autistic pattern, therefore getting a confirmation that I was autistic after doing so much initial research wasn't much of a surprise!

It's daunting to begin explaining my health journey and diagnoses to people, but this is one of the reasons I chose to write about my experiences. I want to help you and the wider population understand the person *beyond* the conditions as well as educating on the symptoms and struggles that come with a disability. I want people to see and understand the reality behind the fancy medical names our invisible battles are given. I want to share my story and my experiences to explain what life can be like for a disabled person. I also want you to know that every single day and every single story looks different.

We can't pre-judge people based on their conditions, their disability, or what they've been through. We also can't pre-judge people based on their lack of labels or diagnoses, because you never know what's going on behind a perfect facade.

That's enough science background for now, but I will be going into more detail about these conditions as they appear in my personal story. First, I want to take you back to the beginning and give you an insight into my life as a whole.

# TWO
# THE REAL ME

To kick-start my health journey, I'd first like to give you some insight into me as a person without any health conditions.

I was born in a small town in England on the 20th of July 2005. I was 6 pounds 7 ounces and actually had a knot in my cord. Apparently, this is a rare birth phenomenon where the baby moves around in the womb so much that a knot is formed and tightened. I was also born with a heart murmur due to a small hole in my heart, which I still have to this day, but doctors marked this as innocent (not affecting me) when I was little, so thankfully we don't have to monitor it any more.

As a toddler, I was extremely outgoing! Throughout my whole life, people have told me that I'm an "old soul" which is very common for autistic women and girls. At age two, I would eat olives at buffets (not a usual choice for a toddler) and confidently chatter with any adults around me—this was the case for most of my early childhood.

I always found it much easier to talk to adults than to the other children my age. I gravitated towards teachers and adults at school and always preferred to spend my play and lunch times in a classroom doing art, writing, or talking to teachers about my work and my hobbies.

This may seem like strange behaviour for a child, but for those of you in the neurodivergent community—specifically autistic people—will hopefully find comfort in relating to some of these traits. If you do, I hope you know that you're not alone and that you don't have to change to fit into what other people your age are doing. It's okay to feel like you're on a slightly different time scale to others or that you're maturing at a different rate (whether that's slower or faster than your peers). Both are perfectly okay, so please don't let comments from other people make you feel you're wrong, because there is no "right" way to grow up!

I've always been an inquisitive and bubbly child, though I was pretty shy around any people I didn't know, especially after starting school. Although I was nervous around other people, I was always animated around my family and my two closest friends (who I am still friends with to this day).

One of my favourite things to do was reading, which I did from around the age of one or two. I've always been "ahead" academically (reading and writing) for my age, which helped me tremendously with my grades in school. I've always preferred to practice reading or writing rather than socialising, but both have their perks I suppose! I'm a huge *Disney* and *Harry Potter* fan, and I love any books related to fantasy, rom-coms (specifically with LGBTQ+ or disability representation) or anything about witches.

Another hobby I've always adored is gymnastics. I did classes as a child, but switched to cheerleading and dance at high-school, which I then coached for a while—oh how times change. In 2022, I returned to my childhood gym and joined an adult gymnastics class, which I now attend every week I'm well enough to… and I absolutely love it.

I also love making art, painting, crafting and doing digital illustrations on my iPad using Procreate. Another lifelong hobby of mine is music. I play the piano (my favourite pieces to play are classical music), guitar, ukulele and I love to sing. I've always written songs for as long as I've been able to talk, and now I record and produce my music using my at-home recording setup. I released my first-ever song "She's Mine" in 2022, which you can listen to on all streaming platforms!

I also spend time walking my dog Lottie in the forests near my house. I always feel better after spending time in nature, and when I'm well enough to move my body I love the gentle exercise too. Going for walks (or wheelchair rolls), picnics, and taking photos of pretty views with my camera are some of my favourite ways to spend time outdoors! I try to get fresh air every day if I am physically able to, because it massively helps my mental health, and I've always felt very connected to nature.

Now… I could tell you about all of my life for *hours*, but I want this book to focus on my health journey and what I've learned, so I'll instead give you a short list of facts about me!

**Fun Facts about Me:**

1. I have a ginger, stripy cat called Jesse. He isn't a fan of hugs, but he always sleeps next to me on a blanket on my bed.
2. I have a puppy called Lottie, who is a very playful salt-and-pepper-coloured labradoodle.
3. Beth is actually my middle name, but I now use it (along with my first name) as my identity online!
4. I played the violin in primary school, but the hobby fizzled out (much to my family's relief).
5. My first name means 'princess' in Russian and 'blooming flower' or 'radiance' in Arabic.

ENEMY FOR A BRAIN

6. Despite my history of gymnastics and being very clumsy, I have yet to break a bone (touch wood), but I've torn and sprained many muscles.
7. I love gaming! My all-time favourite game to play is Minecraft, which I've played for 11 years.
8. I spend most of my free time either reading or writing - I read 140 books last year and I'm aiming for 100 again this year!
9. I meditate and practice yoga every morning and every evening before bed. Stretching makes me feel good—it's low-impact so it doesn't trigger my health issues and it relaxes my fast-paced thoughts.
10. I cannot sleep without reading before I go to bed. I read every single night because it helps me shut off my busy, whirring brain.

The point of this chapter is to give you an insight into me as a person so that before we get stuck into my disabilities and health journey, you see that underneath all the struggles and diagnoses, I am my own person.

I have hobbies, interests, and so many memories and qualities which don't relate to Tourette's, FND, or being autistic. Although I talk about my disabilities a lot online, I do have a life outside of advocacy - but this doesn't invalidate my struggles or make my passion for advocacy any less valid or important.

Having TS does somewhat define me because it changes the way I appear to other people when I'm making noises or twitching. Being autistic changes every single thought I have about the world and how I interact with others, therefore it is a very influential part of my identity. My conditions are something I will live with for the rest of my life, so it makes sense that these are pretty integral parts of my personality.

The reason disabled people like me (who love advocating) seem to talk about being disabled *a lot*, is because our disabilities are a huge part of our identities, just like any other identifier, interest, or difference people may have.

My conditions *do* change my body, mind and the way I go about my days—they make my life pretty damn difficult a lot of the time— but I've slowly learned that this doesn't mean I have to hate them. I don't have to separate or differentiate myself completely from my diagnoses, because they're not something I need to feel ashamed of.

Being different is okay. Sometimes it's tricky, and it causes so many people difficulties, hurt, and pain, and makes them feel alone sometimes. But despite this, being different is arguably a good thing! It makes us interesting and unique. It allows us to think outside of the box and gives us all some individual stories to tell, and diverse perspectives to share.


Now it's time to get stuck into my health story so I can show you —in writing—what my perspective on the world looks like as a disabled and neurodivergent person.

# THREE
## PRIMARY SCHOOL

As a child, I was relatively healthy. My health issues (that I know of now) weren't present until my early teen years, so childhood me was in near-perfect health! I didn't worry too much about fitness, I didn't have seizures or fainting episodes, and I didn't feel exhausted beyond the average level of tiredness. My first struggles actually came in the form of anxiety.

Although this book will focus mostly on physical health, I can't write about chronic illness or disability without mentioning mental health. Our physical and mental health go hand in hand, especially when stress is a trigger for your chronic illness— which has been the case for a lot of my conditions.

I remember being very shy from the age of about seven upwards. I found talking to strangers absolutely terrifying, and I became increasingly fearful of new or loud places. I was still bubbly and chatty to my family and familiar people around me, but it took a while for me to warm up to people after not seeing them for a while.

As I got older, going to school became more difficult due to the social elements beginning to change. When games with rules

ZARA BETH

and equal parts turned into chatting and gossiping, I started to fall behind and stuck out like a sore thumb among my peers.

A vivid memory from primary school had a huge impact on my self-worth and caused me lots of self-doubt and anxiety, even as a child as young as eight. I don't blame the other kids for this, as none of us *truly* know the impact of words or friendship groups at that age, but I want to share this experience in case one of you has been through the same (or similar) feeling of being left out. You are not alone.

If you've ever been made to feel like you're on the outside of the bubble, or that you don't belong inside any bubble at all, please know that you are not the problem. People are different, and hobbies, interests, preferences and personalities are all different, which means that not all of us get along well with each other.

This is even more noticeable during school because we're forced to spend our whole days with kids who may not understand or accept us, which for neurodivergent individuals, can cause many traumatic experiences with being bullied or left out.

∼

As my class moved up into year four (ages 8-9) in primary school, a clear divide developed between friendship groups. We started to mature slightly, kids were deciding who could hang out with who, and the easy dynamic of playing games in the playground disappeared. This may not have been noticeable to many of the other children, but for me, it was incredibly jarring. This change symbolised the transition between not worrying about friendships, to feeling like I was incapable of being accepted.

A clique slowly formed in my class, which was named by the most confident kids in the class as the "cool gang". This may sound harmless and childish to an adult, but as kids, this was the most desirable label to have.

I never considered that I was unlikeable until this moment because I had a few close friends and I hadn't had much trouble with other classmates before... but that all changed with this "clique".

The whole class was invited into this group by the "popular" kids, apart from two children. One of these was me. I was told that I wasn't allowed to join the group, because I wasn't "cool" or likeable enough, which suddenly meant I wasn't allowed to hang out with them any more. I wasn't allowed to play their games, be in their areas of the playground, or even talk to them. This left me feeling incredibly lonely when even my best friend was invited to the clique.

Although this sounds pretty trivial, it affected me a lot. Being excluded created a sense of self-doubt as I was told that I wasn't "cool" enough to be talked to or played with.

That I wasn't good enough.

I wasn't enough.

But, no child should ever be told this, and nor should any child be told that they can't play with others purely because they may think or look slightly different.

Present-tense me knows that I am *enough* and that there are many people who I *can* be good friends with who *do* want to talk to me. I just hadn't found the right people in the school class forced upon us for every single day of our childhoods.

This "cool gang" resulted in me spending a lot of time on my own, or constantly trying to find a way into this untouchable group. Every day I tried to prove myself as good enough to be accepted, but no matter how much I changed or moulded myself to try and fit in, I was never allowed into the clique.

Although this was heartbreaking at the time, it was probably a good thing! It taught me that you need to find your own friends and people because not everybody fits into the same box and *that's okay*. I quickly learned that not all of the people in this group were kind, so I didn't want to be friends with them anyway. I will do a bigger chapter on bullying later on in the book, but I'd like to share a memory from this time in my life too.

~

We were standing in a line in the hallway of my school, waiting to go back into our classroom. I was standing on my own (without a friend to talk to) so I waited and listened to the chatter around me from other children.

Two pupils in front of me were chatting about a party, so I turned to them and listened in. They talked about their birthday which was happening a few weeks later, and had been discussing who they were inviting. They talked about all the invitations they'd made with their parents, and how they'd given them out to everybody in the class. This stuck out in my head as a lie, because I definitely didn't remember receiving an invitation.

I naturally like to believe the best in people, therefore I didn't even consider that my lack of invitation could be intentional. The thought didn't even enter my mind that they could be leaving me out on purpose! (Always assuming the best of people is a great character quality I have thanks to autism and can be useful in many ways, but it's also one that caused me many hurtful misunderstandings).

I tapped one of the children on the shoulder and told them that I hadn't got an invitation, a smile still on my face. They looked at each other, and then looked back at me and laughed. I laughed along because I didn't understand. I couldn't quite read their expressions, and I take things very literally, which can sometimes make me "gullible".

They shot me a look—which I can now infer to be judgement

—and then proceeded to tell me that I wasn't invited to the party. I started to feel upset but tried to hide it. I asked if I could come, trying to redeem the situation, but they didn't take me seriously. There was never a chance of me being invited to the party when I hadn't even been allowed to hang out with them in the playground.

But, the thing that stuck with me was when one of them turned and told me I actually could come to their party. My face lit up and I felt like I finally had a chance. This was it. I was finally being let into this untouchable group.

They then followed this up with, "You can be the bouncy castle" whilst looking my body up and down and laughing with their friend.

This was the first of many comments which have insulted the way I look, although I now know that there was never anything wrong with my body—or my personality for that matter. I was only a child just like every other student in that class, but for one reason or another, I'd been cast out as unworthy of respect or invitations.

I don't write this for sympathy (after years of therapy and a lot of inner confidence work, I have come to terms with the experiences I had in primary school) but rather, to make it known that bullying *does happen*, even in young children. Friendship groups are so incredibly difficult to navigate for children and adults alike, but this is especially difficult for neurodivergent people.

Being an undiagnosed autistic child, I never understood why the other kids didn't like the way I talked, or why I preferred to spend time with the teachers or books rather than playing with other kids. They didn't understand why I enjoyed rules and always reminded the teacher if we had homework due. I didn't understand why I didn't enjoy the same things or why I couldn't pay attention to conversations that weren't about my hobbies, interests or passions. I never understood why I didn't feel like a *real* member of the class.

I felt on the outside.

I now know after talking to so many other neurodivergent adults that this is a very common feeling and experience in this community. We are made to feel like we have to change in order to fit in, which sets us up for failure from a really young age.

It's taken me years to figure out who I am without the influence of other people, and I'm still only a short way into this journey. I have so much to learn and discover about the way my brain works, and I uncover things about myself every single day.

It is not a reflection of you as a person if you're cast out or not accepted by the group you so badly want to fit into. You don't have to change your identity to make yourself more likeable. You don't have to change your interests to match the people around you. If that's the only way you'll fit in with those people, then they are not the right ones for you, and trying hard to fit in with them will never truly make you feel at home.

I've learned that accepting yourself for who you are is more important than staying in any friendship group or earning a higher level of respect from your peers. Being in the bubble or clique isn't as admirable as it seems from the outside, because if you have to change yourself to get in, then you're never going to be accepted as your true self when you do make it in.

My best advice is to be true to yourself, and if people don't like that version of you, then you truly are much better off without them!

I'm now an adult, I don't have a friendship group, and I'm the happiest I've ever been. I learned that I don't want to constantly change myself to fit in, because if I'm not being honest with my true self, then I'm never going to fit into or find the *right* group.

I've wasted too much time trying to change myself to fit in with the people around me, not realising that this will never result in those people liking or accepting me. If you're not your true self, then people will sense this and those friendships will never truly last; it's better to get ahead of the game and try to find the people who accept you when you're *not* changing yourself.

When you're accepted as your fully unmasked, true self, it's much more rewarding than ever being accepted as a "more ideal" or "trendier" version of yourself.

# FOUR
# MY FIRST SIGNS

We noticed my brain worked slightly differently (in a neurological sense) during primary school. My first signs of Tourette's syndrome started to appear, though we didn't know what these were at the time. Only around half of children with Tourette's are officially diagnosed, because tics (involuntary movements and sounds) are often mild which doesn't lead to parents or teachers bringing up any concerns.

My tics didn't cause any noticeable problems until around age fourteen, which is a common time for people with TS to experience a heightened burst of tics.

"It is very common for Tourette syndrome to worsen around the period of puberty. In some cases, this worsening may be such that patients and families feel that the condition began to impact on daily functioning and quality of life only during this period."
-Tourette's Action UK

Not many people know how tics or Tourette's can develop, so I'd like to share my journey of developing tics to give you some insight. Every person's experience looks different, and many people develop tics at different ages, at different speeds, severities, and everybody's tics are different.

If you don't have Tourette's yourself, feel free to use this segment as an educative anecdote so you can learn some of the early signs of tics. If you do have Tourette's, maybe you can relate to this! Or maybe you'll discover that you have experienced some of the same things I have, and had never linked them to TS until now.

~

From around the age of seven, my mum began noticing small twitches in my jaw and my neck that I hadn't realised I was doing. She'd ask me why I was jerking my neck and whether I knew that I was twitching whilst playing on my laptop or watching TV.

I'd subconsciously twitch my jaw and move my head and face all the time, without ever noticing it. I also began clearing my throat and "coughing" or "hiccuping", especially when I was more excited or stressed than usual.

My mum researched about involuntary movements and we discovered that I'd been experiencing **tics**. We asked the GP (general practitioner or primary healthcare doctor in the UK) about these tics, but the investigation didn't go any further and the tics were ruled out as being anxiety-related. I was told that they would gradually disappear as I grew out of them, which is the case for lots of children.

Despite tics being a very common occurrence (and a temporary case for a lot of children), my tics didn't disappear as I got older. In fact, when I later hit puberty, my tics became more out of control than ever. Shortly after my Tourette's diagnosis at age fourteen, my mum and I made the connection that these unexplained childhood hiccups and movements were early signs of my TS.

I recently spoke to a friend with Tourette's and realised another early struggle that went unnoticed was getting my hair cut. Before we knew I had tics, we expected my experience of getting a haircut to be the same as any other child's, but we quickly figured out that this wasn't the case.

Whenever I had to go for a haircut, I'd find myself getting extremely nervous. This was one of the times—along with school, the doctors, the dentist, and meeting strangers—when I started to experience a lot of anxiety. We noticed that along with this anxiety, came hiccups. We didn't understand why, but whenever I got my hair cut I got the hiccups! I had them pretty much every day—any time I was nervous, excited, and even when I didn't realise I was making sounds.

I couldn't stop hiccuping!

We asked the doctor about this, but we never got to the bottom of the mysterious daily hiccups. We just carried on as normal and assumed I had something wrong with my diaphragm causing me to hiccup more than usual.

These hiccups were soon followed by twitching. When I'd go to the hairdressers and begin hiccuping, my shoulders would twitch upwards and I couldn't keep my head still. This made it impossible for me to sit still in the chair and made it very difficult for the hairdresser to do her job and cut my hair evenly.

This happened a few times before my mum decided to instead cut my hair at home herself. To this day—though we now know my "hiccups" and twitches are tics—my mum still trims my hair at home, saving me the stress and embarrassment of trying (and failing) to keep still while sitting in the hairdresser's chair.

Another symptom I began experiencing at this age was circulatory issues.

From the age of about eight or nine, I'd struggle to shower due to not being able to stand for long without my legs developing a rash which looked like neon-orange hives. We tried different shampoos, conditioners, soaps and I even tried using hypo-allergenic products designed for sensitive skin... but none of these worked.

A few years ago, after being introduced to the symptoms of POTS at a specialist clinic (more on this in Chapter 21), a doctor told me I suffered from Orthostatic Intolerance, which can cause blood pooling in the form of rash-like marks along the feet and legs after standing. This made all the childhood "allergy rashes" make sense!

I also struggled with my circulation in school because I felt dizzy every time I went from sitting on the carpet to standing with everybody else. My hands would go numb and tingly more than usual, and every time we sat on the hall floor for primary school assemblies, I'd notice my legs went completely numb after sitting cross-legged.

I remember trying to stand up with my class and realising that my legs were numb with pins and needles—when I tried to walk, I couldn't feel my toes touching the ground and I tripped over my own feet.

Nobody else around me ever experienced this so it was always confusing and inconvenient, but we didn't get answers until many years later.


The last struggle I want to mention here is how early in my life I began experiencing sensory issues. I will go into more detail about this in Chapter 27 (maybe I will write a whole other book on autism one day!) but, since getting my autism diagnosis, I've spent hours thinking about my childhood. I've thought over events, feelings, friendships, and pretty much every aspect of my world from earlier in my life, and I have uncovered so many traits which weren't picked up on at the time. One of these was sensory issues.

I wasn't a particularly picky eater as a child, but I was very specific about certain rules around food. I wouldn't eat anything that had mixed with other foods—for example, if my peas touched the beans on my plate, or if my fish fingers came into contact with my vegetables. I also didn't like the texture of squishy things, the consistency of yoghurt, and so many other textures or materials which don't involve food.

I struggled to brush my teeth due to the feeling of the bristles rubbing my teeth and the cold water hurting my gums. I also struggled immensely with clothing. I remember spending hours each weekend trying to choose what to wear, trying on every single item and ripping it back off as it felt "wrong" on my body. My leggings were too tight and made me feel trapped, my tops didn't have the right texture, jumpers were a complete sensory nightmare, and the list goes on. I didn't wear socks, and if I was forced to wear them for school or occasions, I'd wear them inside out so I couldn't feel the uneven seams throughout the day.

I couldn't explain why, but these things caused me so much distress that I'd become irritable, sad, tearful and sometimes completely panicked.

These were early signs of autism and OCD.

At the time, I thought I was being inconvenient or silly, or that I had no real reason to feel the amount of distress as I did from these things. I felt confused and didn't understand why these seemingly "simple" tasks were so difficult for me when they were easy for everybody else.

A lot of people who are late diagnosed with mental health struggles, autism or ADHD, have spent the majority of their lives trying to understand why they struggle. Why everything feels more difficult for them than for neurotypical people.

We're left questioning whether it's because we're not focused enough, or smart enough, or whether we're the problem... but you are not! *We* are not the problem.

Being late-diagnosed, or not having appropriate understanding and support, can leave neurodivergent people feeling abandoned, and like we're a problem that needs to be fixed. As a community, we've all felt a sense of not belonging at some point in our lives, which has led to so many of us doubting ourselves as people.

Having sensory issues, anxiety, depression, OCD, or being autistic or ADHD, does not make you difficult or any less worthy of a person. Having struggles doesn't mean you aren't deserving of patience or the same opportunities as other people. Not being able to do "simple" daily tasks does not make you a failure. And being neurodivergent is not a problem that needs to be fixed or erased.

Although society often depict these neurological realities as deficits or problems, neurotypical people need to understand that neurodivergent people are just as worthy and capable as them. We just work in a slightly different way that isn't widely accommodated for or accepted in society! This lack of accessibility and accommodations available to support neurodivergent individuals is the true deficit.

# FIVE
# SECONDARY SCHOOL

The transition between primary school (ages 3-11 in the UK) and secondary school (ages 11-16 in the UK) is difficult for everybody, but as a neurodivergent child, this turned my entire world upside down.

Suddenly, games in the playground with rules and physical activity turned into sitting and gossiping at tables, one teacher for the whole year turned into five different teachers per day, and one classroom turned into an entire school to navigate. The corridors were loud, there were a thousand students rather than only two hundred, you had to pay for your own food at the canteen, and you could eat lunch wherever you liked in the school.

Every rule and normality from primary school was suddenly ripped away, sending me into a spiral of unknown territory filled with constant change and decisions. This is where my anxiety hit an all-time high as I struggled to cope with the change physically, mentally and socially.

Change is inevitable in life, but it's also something that most neurodivergent people struggle to cope with. If you're like me, then you'll love routines and knowing where you'll be at every minute of every day. I like planning my days meticulously to give myself structure even on my rest days: this clears my head space and gives me a more productive and calm mindset. In my experience, struggling to cope with routine changes was a common autistic trait that I resonated a lot with during my undiagnosed school years.

However, I understand that not everybody's mind works the same. In fact, every single one works differently! We all have our own individual ways of functioning, and this is known as **neurodiversity**.

Even after a few months of settling in, I still felt anxious and was constantly on edge at school. I became upset and frustrated beyond "normal" or "reasonable" levels whenever there were unexpected changes to plans or environments. Whether it was a surprise assembly, a substitute teacher in one of my classes, a spontaneous maths test I didn't have time to plan for, or something as simple as people sitting in different seats at the lunch tables… every single change made my head feel like it was exploding.

Lunchtime quickly became one of my most dreaded times of day, as it involved standing in groups and chatting. I didn't understand the topics being spoken about or the expressions people were pulling. I didn't know when people were making fun of me or when they were being serious. I didn't understand why friends constantly spoke badly about others and then proceeded to smile and chat to those same girls. It was a social minefield, and it felt like I'd been thrown in at the deep end.

I think everybody struggles with cliques and friendships to some extent in school because teenagers can be mean! Girls are especially "bitchy" during these few secondary school years, and groups frequently split up and change as new friendships form and old ones are lost.

My experience with friendship groups was never consistent or reliable. I found myself being passed between groups, always trying hard to find a place which didn't make me feel unwelcome. I found it incredibly draining to keep up a persona to match the around me and to keep up with topics of conversation which didn't naturally spark my interest.

Small talk doesn't come naturally to me, and if I don't have a particular interest in a topic then I can find it hard to engage with the conversation since I can't info-dump or use my own experiences as a baseline. I often felt like I wasn't on the same planet as other classmates, meaning I frequently spaced out of conversations or laughed along for the sake of "looking the part" even when I didn't understand the joke.

I'm sharing my perspective to give you an insight into my teenage brain, but this definitely isn't what people saw from the outside. My early struggles were invisible to the outside world unless I chose to show somebody my true self or talked to someone about my feelings. However, in my case, I never spoke up. My instinct told me to hide away and bottle up my thoughts so that I wouldn't be judged. I didn't want to create a problem by admitting that I was struggling.

(If you're reading this and you can relate, please know that this is never the case! Please speak up if you feel like this, because I can assure you that you are not creating a problem. You are not a problem because you're struggling. You deserve help and support, and you will be able to get this when you're surrounded by the right people.)

I squashed down all of my feelings in an attempt to mask any signs of being different; I just wanted to fit in and be accepted.

And for a while, it worked. I was a good student with straight-A grades, I attended every single after-school club, I was on the hockey team, and the netball team, I did dance and cheerleading, I was an English ambassador, mentor, I was in the choir, I was a form monitor, I volunteered for every single open day and event that I could. I got the top grades in a lot of my classes, and never got anything wrong on weekly spelling tests. The list goes on.

I was such a busy teen at the ages of eleven to fourteen that I didn't have any space for extra thoughts. I kept every single day filled with tasks and activities and spent a lot of time studying or doing homework to perfect my grades and ensure I kept up the 100% exam expectations. I know my teachers wouldn't *really* have been mad at me if I'd gotten a 96% instead of a 99%, but to me, this felt like a huge failure. It felt like I'd failed at the one thing I was consistently good at and praised for.

This pressure was also echoed by my classmates when we'd get our test results back and the whole class would ask each other what score they'd got. Many people would turn to me and ask, but before I could even answer somebody would usually interrupt to say "of course she got 100%, why are you even asking?" which made me feel like I'd failed if I got anything less.

I found my place as the goody-two-shoes, straight-A student who all the teachers knew and praised for being a top student… and for a while I was good at it. It was stressful, and I still struggled with all my social interactions and with my mental health behind the scenes, but I kept up this perfect, quiet, shy student appearance for years.

While this acted as a survival mechanism for a while, this was detrimental to my mental health, and as of recent years, it eventually led to immense physical and mental burnout, along with the start of my chronic illnesses.

Behind the mask I'd perfected, I was struggling with severe anxiety and depression by the age of twelve. In year eight of secondary school (age 12-13) I began having panic attacks which quickly became daily occurrences. They began interrupting my lessons, my friendships, my break times and pretty much every aspect of my life. During this time, not even my parents knew what was going on because I was so afraid to tell anybody due to the fear of being judged—even though people in my life were caring and understanding.

Because I felt like I couldn't tell my friends or family what was going on, I eventually asked a trusted member of staff at my school if I could have a pass to get out of lessons, which they approved. I didn't have to tell my mum, and nobody would know except from my subject teachers, so this seemed like a miracle at the time!

I used this pass nearly every single lesson for the next few months and every day for the next few years. I frequently fell behind in class because I'd be too busy trying to regulate my breathing, staring at the too-loudly ticking clock and planning escape routes every second of the day. I'd be in tears multiple times through every school day, and hiding in the bathrooms whenever I had to socialise at lunch time. I left my lessons to stand in the corridor and hyperventilate as another panic attack set in, and still, I hid this from everybody I possibly could.

When you're in the midst of anxiety and depression, you can't think clearly or see past the fuzzy state you're trapped in. It's hard to see the point in reaching out when you're convinced it will only make people hate you anyway. You feel like nobody in the world understands, and that telling people would only draw attention to yourself when the only thing you want is to disappear.

Mental illness is exhausting, it's draining. It takes everything you have physically and mentally until you're a fraction of yourself.

I felt incredibly lonely in years seven, eight and nine. I had close friends, but they didn't truly understand me, and I had to change myself to ensure I fitted in with their aesthetic or social expectations. I had good grades, but I spent all of my energy trying to keep them up under the immense pressure of maintaining the winning streak. I seemed quiet and hard-working, but underneath I was slowly drowning in my own pressure and worries.

Mental illness can seem invisible to people looking in, and it can happen to anybody. You don't have to come from a traumatic background to struggle with anxiety; you don't need to be poor to struggle with depression. Anybody at any age, from any background and upbringing can suffer with their mental health.

It can be especially tricky for high-flying students or successful working people to open up about mental illness because they feel they have a persona to keep up with. They have an impenetrable, high-achieving reputation that they've curated, and for many adults, a mental illness may feel like a failure or a weakness. They may be afraid to admit that they're struggling because they don't want to seem vulnerable or inferior. They may fear people will treat them differently if they open up about their struggles, so they stay quiet.

Much like I did as a teenager, many people battling mental illness feel like they need to hide or bottle up their struggles so they don't appear to be weak, but this shouldn't be the case. We should feel like whoever we are, however old we are, and whatever background we come from, we have a safe place to ask for help. We should feel accepted and understood. We should feel validated. We should feel like we can get help without being judged or treated like we're less capable purely because we struggle with a mental battle.

Mental health isn't understood as much as it needs to be. We talk about mental health a lot more at present, but people are still being missed. I know individuals who have been missed by the healthcare system or who couldn't get access to the help they needed for their mental health, and they have suffered, or even died as a result of this.

I myself have struggled with the dark sides of depression; the side people never see. I spent years of my early teens wishing I could disappear, and not seeing the point in living any more. I shut everybody out in order to hide what I was going through, and I became so resentful of myself that I thought there was no place for me in the world.

I looked successful, hard-working, smiley, and like any other teen from the outside, but on the inside, I was falling apart.

Suicide is a real threat that people are afraid to talk about or admit responsibility for. Suicide is more common than any of us would like to accept, and the only time this is acknowledged is when it's too late.

When people reach out for accommodations or support—whether it's for their physical or mental health—they are often redirected or shut down, which leads to them feeling dismissed and alone. Due to the lack of staff and resources, healthcare in the UK usually only offers mental health services to those who are in crisis or who are most at risk of harm. This leaves so many people without support or any help with their struggles.

Asking for help is often seen as inconvenient or annoying by people who don't understand the true impact accommodations can have. But these accommodations save lives. Talking about—and understanding—mental illness saves lives. Reaching out and offering support to people early on, rather than realising that you could've done more later, saves lives.

As a society, there is so much more we can do to help people battling mental illness, yet a lot of people don't want to go out of their way to make this possible because they see it as an inconvenience to their lives. They don't want to slow down or get distracted from their own life because somebody else has asked for help, so they direct people onto others and wipe their hands clean of the task or responsibility. But doing this and being a bystander means that so many disabled, neurodivergent or mentally ill people slip under the radar and don't get the support they need to be happy or healthy.

So please, reach out to people and check in on them even if they seem to have everything put together because you never know what's really going on behind the scenes.

If you have struggled with mental illness yourself, you're struggling to reach out or you relate to my experiences, then please ask for help when you need it. You are not a burden, and anybody who makes you feel like you are is not worth your time, because you are worth so much more.

I wish I'd reached out sooner when I was struggling at age twelve. I wish I could go back and hug my younger self and tell her that everything will be okay, and one day I will be confident voicing my struggles and asking for help whenever needed. I can't go back in time, but I can say to everybody reading this, that there truly is hope.

You are worthy. You are important. You are lovable. And you deserve so much.

# SIX
# BULLYING

We've talked about bullying in this book already, but I'm afraid it's time for yet another conversation. I'm not sure why I was bullied for so many years, but I can presume that people singled me out because of my awkward nature. Or maybe it wasn't anything particular at all! Sometimes kids are mean just because they can be, and you happen to be in the wrong place at the wrong time. Sometimes kids are going through difficult things which they don't know how to process, leading them to lash out at others around them.

Neither of these are excuses for bullying somebody, but they may give you some insight into why people are negative towards others and show you that it's not your fault if you fall victim to bullying. Being bullied does not mean *you* should change, and it doesn't indicate that anything was ever "wrong" with you in the first place.

What I'm about to share is a three-year span of bullying I experienced in secondary school—which has stayed with me and can still affect my confidence to this day.

Besides the mental health struggles already developing in

secondary school, another significant part of my life was bullying. Like many other neurodivergent people have experienced, I was bullied at primary and secondary school. This occurred before my tics became severe, and before my health issues became noticeable. People singled me out due to the way I looked (though there was never anything wrong with my appearance!) and the fact I never quite fit in.

As we've discussed in earlier chapters, I silently struggled with friendships and socialising from a young age. I was oddly good at making random acquaintances—I'd always find somebody to play with at play centres or the park—but when it came to real, deep friendships or social groups, I couldn't grasp or understand why I kept being left out. *Why I couldn't just be like my peers?*

This ultimately led to trying my absolute hardest to fit in. I unconsciously morphed myself into whichever friendship group I had at the time, therefore in years seven to eleven (and even part of college) my fashion, texting style, attitude and personality significantly changed based on who I was friends with. This wasn't intentional and a lot of the time I didn't notice I was doing it at all!

After I learned about autistic traits over the last few years, I recognised this behaviour to be 'masking'. I can now identify this and kindly catch myself any time I begin trying to blend in again. I've always struggled to find out *who* I am without trying to impress or blend in with other people around me, but I'll talk more on this later.

~

I remember being terrified during the teenage years of my life. Terrified to go to school, terrified in the corridors, in the canteen, during PE lessons, when walking home and even when I got home—as I'd be alone in my bedroom with my anxious brain.

Thanks to the wonderful creation of the mobile phone, I also brought the torment of bullying home from school with me every night. Although social media has its positives (such as me writing this book now), it certainly has negatives too.

I've found huge positives in reaching all the people who follow me and being able to tell my story. We can find community, friends, connect with people we never could've met without the internet, and we can learn pretty much any skill with a video tutorial. The internet is very useful in many ways, but it's also one of the biggest threats, especially to young and impressionable teenagers.

Cyberbullying is a real and very frightening thing to go through; it isolates you and often forces you into silence using manipulative threats of posting photos or revealing something you don't want people to know about. Cyberbullying can happen to anybody, at any time, and it's even more prevalent nowadays because most teenagers have their own phones. We have portable devices in our pockets which allow anybody in the world to send us a comment or a message anonymously, giving them the ability to say horrible things without ever showing their face. This is the danger many children are now facing at increasingly young ages.

I've experienced in-person, online, verbal, and physical bullying over the years, and I can assure you that none of these are pleasant things to go through.

My experience started with pretty harmless comments. Girls would reply to my Snapchat stories saying things like "I hate your room, it looks shit" and seemingly meaningless comments. However, these things still hurt to hear as a twelve-year-old.

When you're young, it can be difficult to differentiate between generalised comments and outright personal attacks, but it's never nice to hear insults or negative things about yourself regardless. Over time, the comments became progressively more targeted and much more personal.

I don't wish for sympathy or pity (really, I'm okay!) and I now understand that none of this was my fault, but I do know other children, teens and adults may be experiencing this too.

Bullying happens everywhere, at every age, in any situation. Bullies exist online, in person, in schools, in workplaces, and sometimes even in families. I'm lucky to have had the support of my family and my school, which led to the bullying eventually ending, but this isn't always the case for others. We need to be more aware of similar experiences that are often overlooked, because it can feel impossible for victims of bullying to speak out —especially if they're being threatened by the people targeting them.

If you know somebody who is being bullied, you know of someone who is bullying others, or you're being bullied yourself, then *please* reach out to someone you can trust. Whether it's a teacher, your school, your family, parents, siblings, friends, or even a helpline, there is *always* somebody you can go to. Things can get better if you find people you can trust, so please try to remember that this is not your fault and it is *never* okay for people to be unkind to other human beings.

It's time to share my perspective as a victim of bullying through a short anecdote. This part of my life shaped how I interact and respond to negativity, so it is an important part of my health journey. I truly believe that I wouldn't have coped so well with my health challenges or be as open-minded as I have been with my diagnoses if it weren't for my earlier experiences with negativity.

Although it was difficult to cope with at the time, I'm thankful I now have the skills to let negative comments wash over me and to always pride myself on who I am away from other people's comments. Knowing your own worth can make a world of a difference.

~

After the text messages progressed to more hurtful words, a group of girls added me to a group chat where multiple people sent photos and screenshots of me. They sent nasty comments about my appearance, called me slurs and invited their friends to the group so they could join in on the "fun" of mocking me.

It was mortifying! It felt like my life was over. *If I couldn't slip through secondary school unnoticed, then how was I ever going to be happy? How would I ever survive in the real world if I couldn't blend in enough to escape the girls in my year?*

But unfortunately, it didn't stop there. The online comments became more frequent and the private messages became spam calls or video chats—which I never answered. I'd watch calls light up my screen as panic stuck through me, counting to ten and waiting for the call to stop ringing. The insults also spread from targeting me alone, to targeting my entire friendship group. They called us all "a group of gays" which, looking back on it, ironically turned out to be quite true, though it was used as an insult back then.

Going to school can be a difficult part of any teenager's life, but it became my version of torture. On top of the rising anxiety and daily panic attacks sent my way, the bullying became more physical too. I remember dreading PE classes every single week because I had to run laps in front of the girls who openly mocked and ridiculed me. I'd take my turn to run while they sat on the sidelines laughing and pointing at me, imitating the way my cheeks and face jiggled when I ran. I didn't have a particularly sporty or athletic body as a young teen, which meant I wasn't naturally good at running. The girls took advantage of my normal, human appearance and caused me to despise it for years.

You'll be happy to hear that at age nineteen, I have now overcome my hatred of running and I took it up again a few years ago before my health became too limiting. My face and body still jiggle, but that is not because I'm the centre of teen girls' jokes… it's because I am human.

I love exercising! When I'm well enough and my body cooperates, it's freeing and enjoyable (especially when the weather is nice), so I'm grateful to have overcome this part of my childhood and teenage life. The thing that caused so much ridiculing for many years actually turned out to be a source of freedom; how ironic.


But alas, PE was just *one* class I felt unsafe in. My worst sources of fear and hatred for school were the corridors and the playground: the dreaded social areas of school. The breeding grounds for all friendships, breakups, drama, and in my case, bullying.

Every time I waited in the corridor for my lessons to start—patiently standing outside the door before being let into the classroom—I'd be on constant high-alert and scanning the corridor for "those girls". If I saw one girl in particular, I'd hide or run to the toilets to escape a confrontation, even if it made me late to class. However, I didn't only feel unsafe on social media and in school; I began to feel unsafe on my walk home from school too.

I walked the same route home every single day: down a dirt track, round the field and to a river, which I crossed on the lower bridge to get to the road. There was a much taller bridge parallel to the one I walked on. It was probably thirty feet higher, the width of a road (with pavements) and had massive arches underneath. A big bridge.

I'd always enjoyed my walk home because it felt safe. It was a breath of fresh air, an escape from all the daily distress. My walk to school gave me ten minutes of nature and harmless chit-chat with a friend, but this soon shattered.

After school one day, I was walking home across the small bridge when my friend and I felt pebbles and plastic bottles falling off the top of the bridge. Because we were on the small, low bridge—which was only wide enough for one person to cross at a time—I couldn't see who was on the big bridge above us, therefore we assumed it was troublemaker boys and carried on with our days. However, when this occurrence became weekly, twice a week, every few days, and then every day... we started to question what was happening. Nobody else had things thrown at them, so why did we?


A few weeks later, I finally saw the people throwing things after being hit on the head for the fourth time that week, this time by a weighty rock which left a mark—looking back, this could have been quite dangerous!

My friend and I heard laughing from the top of the big bridge and, as usual, we sprinted across our small bridge as fast as possible, in fear of being hit again. After making it across, we noticed that the people throwing things were the same ones who sent me messages and mocked me in PE class.

I continued fearing my walk home every day and frequently ran as fast as I could in the hopes of escaping things being thrown by the "popular kids" on the top bridge. I hadn't picked up on the severity of these experiences until one of my best friends at the time (who frequently walked home with me) voiced how she didn't want to walk home with me anymore because she feared for her own safety.

This broke my heart, as I knew I was putting her in harm's way just by associating with me on my walk home. She told her parents, and I told my mum, then somehow (I can't remember every detail as this was nearly seven years ago!) we got the school involved and the rock-throwing stopped, thankfully before anybody was seriously hurt.

I always believed I was safe once I'd passed the river and said goodbye to my friends, but as I walked home one day, I heard laughing and giggling from somewhere I couldn't see. Assuming it was other school kids walking back to their houses, I put my headphones back in and walked along as usual. Later that night, I was sent multiple videos of me walking home from different angles which were posted on the girls' social media stories. They knew where I lived, knew my route home, and I was later followed all the way to my street while they laughed until I ran through my front door. I felt incredibly trapped. I was still only thirteen.

This happened a few times again, therefore I decided to walk the long thirty-minute route to school instead of the ten-minute path over the bridge. I had to leave for school a lot earlier, but it seemed to solve the problem. I actually arrived to school at quarter to eight each morning—despite classes starting at quarter to nine—to remove any risk of seeing other students on my way to school.

This is when I first confided in my favourite teacher, who had been incredibly welcoming and offered to listen when I was upset. I chatted to her nearly every day, and those moments became some of my most fond memories of secondary school.

Another experience that I will always remember happened during lesson change-over. In the corridor, there were people were everywhere, shoulder-to-shoulder, cramming through doors and shoving people to the side with their elbows to get through the onslaught of pupils. I wasn't very tall, so I often got lost in the crowd and pushed further into the barrel of people. It was like being swept along by a tidal wave.

These scary, crowded corridors are a vivid memory that I know a lot of anxious people reading this may relate to. Other students found the hustle and bustle exciting and funny, whereas I only felt claustrophobic and panicked. I eventually got permission to leave lessons early to avoid the "corridor crush" and this helped immensely!

On this particular day, I managed to push through the crowds to the outside and found a stationary spot against the wall, breathing a sigh of relief as I escaped another near-panic attack. But, as soon as I put my guard down, I felt a tug from somebody. I whipped my head around to see a person I feared most: one of the girls who bullied me.

She pushed me against the wall so quickly and violently that my head smacked against the hard surface, making my head even fuzzier than it already felt in the crowded environment. She was laughing about how she'd sneaked up on me, making fun of my scared expression. Her friends laughed along, but I like to believe they didn't quite agree with her; she was the only one who was ever physical with me, though that doesn't make the other girls' comments any less damaging.

The three of them trapped me against the wall, surrounding me with their comments and laughter. I felt like a rabbit in a cage. Except this rabbit is in a cage, and it's in a testing facility and it's about to be murdered and has only just figured out its fate.

I don't remember how exactly I did this or where I found the strength to fight back, but I squeezed out from in between the group and sprinted down the busy corridor. They caught up to me multiple times, but I pushed through people as fast as I could, cutting them off behind me. The main girl followed me all the way through the crowd, down two corridors and I genuinely feared what would happen after she finally caught up to me. I ran straight past the queue of people waiting to go into my maths lesson, but instead of joining them, I continued running even though I knew it'd make me late to my lesson. I didn't want my classmates to witness me being picked on or laughed at.

Being a classic "teachers-pet" student, I ran straight to my head of year's office, dodging the crowd as fast as I could with tears streaming down my face. This teacher briefly knew about some messages sent to me earlier that year, so she already knew I'd been bullied in the past. I knew I could talk to her, so I went to her office and the girls stopped followed me when they realised where I was running.

I'm forever grateful that I decided to speak up that day and ask for help. At the beginning, I found it nearly impossible to report any bullying because of the threats thrown at me about what they'd tell everybody if I went to the teachers and "told on them".

Please know that if you're being bullied, blackmailed, or you feel unsafe reaching out for help, it will get better. It feels so scary in the moment and it can feel like the last thing you want to do is ask for help, but there will always be someone you can talk to. There is always something that can be done, so please don't let yourself suffer in silence.


After calming down my breathing, my teacher gave me a hug, some tissues and talked through what had happened. Time and time again, I told her about the trouble I was experiencing with people in my year and she worked with my mum to report the bullying and keep it under control as much as we could. My experiences lasted over six years in both primary and secondary school, but (much to my relief) the main bully from my secondary school was expelled a year after this incident, leaving me to walk the corridors more freely, focus on my studies and prioritise my worsening mental health.

After that, I didn't hear from any of the girls until a few years ago when my TikTok videos started going viral. When I'd gained just over 400,000 followers, a message popped up from the main girl who'd given me trouble in secondary school, and she apologised for what she'd done. She asked to be friends, but I thanked her for the apology and politely declined. I now know my worth and will only accept friendship from people who appreciate me for who I've always been, before and after my online presence.

The bullying did end after this, and I haven't experienced bullying in a classroom ever since—though I have had my fair share of hate comments online in the past few years.

My experience with peers at school was *far* from easy or smooth-sailing. I jumped between more friendship groups than I can remember, and became the subject of many jokes, but the reason my story is important is so we can spread the word that bullying is never, *ever* okay.

My high school self was deserving of so much better, but I was too afraid to ask for help until the lowest breaking point, and even then, the problem didn't disappear right away. It took time and so much trust to be built before I felt safe, secure and happy again. But I did get here!

If you experience anything which makes you feel unsafe, unhappy, unsatisfied with yourself, or you're made to feel not good enough... it is **not** okay. This behaviour should be reported and dealt with, and you deserve to be given the best chance at having a successful school life. You do not exist to withstand the abuse of others, nor are you here to merely hide from people who threaten you. You are deserving of love, and care, and true friendship. You deserve to feel safe and appreciated.

There are helplines linked at the back of this book, so please feel free to use these if you are struggling and are in need of support.

One of the main reasons I survived during my school years was my form teacher. Even when I felt unable to share what I was going through with most people around me, I had one person who I could tell everything. She comforted me and made sure to do everything possible to fix the problem. She sat with me for hours on end, problem solving and playing guessing games when words were too difficult for me to truly admit. She pulled me from a pretty dark and hopeless place, and allowed me the opportunity to grow into the person I am today.

I know she'll want to read this and support me just like she did the day she took me on as her student, so I want to say thank you for everything. Those words don't feel like enough, but they're all I can share here, so it'll have to do.

It's not always easy to talk to teachers, family, or even friends, but trust me when I say there is always a way to get support. Whether it's helplines, safeguarding staff at school, an online friend, counselling service, or even using online communities where like-minded people can come together and share their experiences. There is always a place for you to open up and get support.

Trust that you will be okay, that things will get better, and that change *can* happen. Try to embrace it when it does.

# SEVEN
# SETTLING IN

After the bullying died down, I settled into a routine as much as possible for the next few years of school. I had friendship groups —although I still struggled and swapped between them quite often—and I was able to focus on my work, my after-school clubs and my lessons better than ever before.

Year nine was my best year in secondary school, because I'd just moved halves of the year following the bullying and a big friendship break-up. Although the change of moving to a new set of classes was jarring, it gave me a start fresh without having to move to an entirely different school and deal with new buildings and teachers too.

When I moved to the other half of my year group, I also moved form classes—which in the UK is your registration class at the beginning of every day. After building such a great bond with my RE teacher, I moved to her form class! This meant that every day, instead of having to visit in my free time or during lunch periods, I'd see her every morning before classes.

This helped me an incredible amount and made me feel like I had a safe space in the school. Every morning, I felt a sense of calm wash over me when talking to the group of girls who sat at the front of my form classroom. We all became friends during these times of the day—though I didn't really hang out with them at all outside of form time—and we quickly became my teacher's "girl band" which I absolutely loved.

Everything felt settled for a while! I tried to ignore the panic attacks I still had on lots of days, and I gradually felt more confident using my pass to get out of lessons when everything felt overwhelming.

However, something I still struggled *a lot* with was school assemblies. When sitting in the hall, I felt trapped—I suffered with so much anxiety that I kept having to escape and run out of the room. People would always look as I slipped down the sides of the chair-lined hall, and this upset me even more—I just wanted to blend in, but my brain wouldn't cooperate.

My form teacher helped by letting me sit at the edge of the hall, instead of sitting in my place alphabetically, which meant that I could easily get up and leave whenever I needed to. Later, when my tics worsened, I stopped going to assemblies altogether, and this helped reduce my anxiety too.

If you also struggle with anxiety, or have any other reasons for needing to leave assemblies because of your disability, sitting in an isle seat may be a good adaptation to ask for.

Halls full of students can be extremely intimidating for somebody who's autistic or has anxiety, and having a disability can be difficult to manage when you can't quickly escape the room, so this could be helpful for many people currently in education.

∾

In late 2019 (during year nine of secondary school) I noticed something beginning to change. Remember the jaw tic I'd had since being around seven years old? Well, it began to happen more. And more. And more, and more, and *even more.*

It had never gone away as a child, but because it was mild, I hadn't noticed it much amongst all the other things I'd been concentrating on. The twitches didn't interrupt my life significantly or cause me pain, so I didn't really give much thought to them. It was just something weird my body did sometimes.

But... it suddenly started to happen a lot more frequently, which caught me really off guard. I'd notice it in lessons, while walking to school, at home, and even while I was busy trying to do other things like gaming or reading. Wherever I was, whatever I was doing, my jaw and neck would twitch without me wanting it to.

This confused me, because at the time, I had no idea what was happening or why it was becoming so out of control. I began to experience a lot of muscle cramps in my shoulders, and eventually developed severe pain down my neck and back from the sheer amount of times my head would twitch throughout the day.

My throat clearing tic increased in frequency too; I'd often clear my throat during lessons which made me feel like everybody was watching me. They weren't, of course—because throat clearing or coughing is a very normal noise to hear in a school—but because I was a quiet teen with anxiety, I hated making *any* noise in the silent classrooms.

I eventually worked up some courage and talked to my mum about the neck pain, crying and holding my neck. I explained how the childhood tic had started again and was even worse than before. She reassured me that it'd probably quieten down soon when I was less stressed. And although this was usually the case, this time the tic didn't ease off.

I began making louder coughing noises in classes, and in addition to the neck, jaw and facial twitches, my arm began jutting out to the side uncontrollably. It felt like somebody was moving my body like a puppet. I couldn't stop it and I didn't know when it was going to happen—my body just did it.

A few people began to notice the tics so I started trying to hide them. I wanted to avoid any possible reason to make people laugh at me—I knew how mean teenagers could be, so I wasn't taking any chances.

As I developed a few more twitches and some squeaky, sniffle sounds, it became harder and harder to hide them. I frequently used my panic-attack pass to leave my lessons, but I started to use it even more when I felt my tics getting worse. I'd leave my lessons when the room fell silent or when I couldn't stop "hiccuping" and twitching my neck. I'd often have panic attacks caused by the sheer stress of trying to conceal these new and unexplained tics.

Eventually, I developed a whistle tic which was the loudest and most noticeable tic I'd had yet. It drew the attention of anybody nearby and sounded a little like catcalling somebody or a twitter notification. I was mortified.

To present day me, a tic like this would be a mild one! But back then, it seemed like the end of the world. I didn't know how I was going to hide it, and I couldn't imagine anything worse than people looking at or noticing me. My ultimate goal was to blend in and just survive school, so these noises and movements made me feel incredibly exposed.

For a few months, I found a temporary "solution". One of my friends at the time had anxiety tics, which the entire year group knew about and had gotten used to. People laughed at her when she first joined our school, but they quickly acclimatised to her making noises in classes or randomly screaming during assemblies.

She was one of the first people to notice my tics, and told me that she experiences the exact same thing—which at the time I didn't want to believe. I didn't want to accept that my tics were a "real problem" that might not go away quickly. I didn't want to believe that I truly was different, so I continued to hide them.

This friend sat next to me in one of my science classes and very quickly became my saving grace. Every time I whistled and quickly tried to disguise that it was me, people just looked towards my friend and then got on with their work. They assumed it was her making the noises, which they'd already accepted and gotten over! We both acknowledged this, and she said I could blame any of my loud tics on her because people wouldn't ask questions that way—I was so thankful!

I began to make louder whistles, or even shouts which sounded halfway between a scream and a word, but everybody in that class thought it was my friend next to me. When the people in front of us turned around and asked if it was me making the noise, we quickly told them it was just her tics and my heart calmed down again until the next time.

This was really helpful because it gave me time to get used to my tics without people in that class judging me. It enabled me to hide a little longer, which at the time seemed like the only option. This friend also became one of my closest companions, and I'm really grateful to have had her to talk to during this tricky period.

Nowadays, I don't think I *needed* to hide my tics back then, and I wouldn't ever hide them like this now because I've accepted them as a part of me. But at first, when I had no explanation as to why they were happening, I really rejected the idea of my tics.

As months passed, my tics became even more noticeable. I missed so many lessons due to leaving class that I'd fallen a little behind. My mind was so distracted that I couldn't concentrate any more. Every lesson was a constant challenge to hold back the movements and noises, meaning I had no brain space left to learn and concentrate on what was being taught. But despite this, I still managed to hide all of this struggle for months—both from my family and from most of the people at school.

That was until one day when we had a surprise assembly…

I'd usually find a way out of assemblies—either by going to the toilet and staying there the whole time, or asking to sit out and stay with my form tutor—but sometimes the teachers held surprise assemblies where all students were escorted to the hall mid-way through a lesson.

On this occasion, I filed in with the other pupils and sat in my seat at the end of the row, ensuring I still had an escape. I remember feeling anxious to the point of feeling slightly ill. Anxiety is never a nice feeling and can often present in very physical sensations such as feeling nausea or chest pains.

I remember tracing the edges of the huge floor-length curtains with my eyes to distract myself until the assembly was over. I couldn't look forward at the projector screen or the teacher who was speaking, because I'd suddenly be hyper-aware of the two hundred people in the hall and I'd start to panic. But my anxiety wasn't the thing that sent me into full panic, this time it was my tics.

I'd never experienced a feeling like it before; my whole body felt tingly, like I had energy running underneath my skin that felt like it was going to explode. My chest felt tight and fuzzy, and my arms felt like they were physically buzzing with energy vibrations. It felt like I'd had ten gallons of caffeine and couldn't sit still.

These feelings worsened when I tried not to tic or move my head obviously enough for the people to notice behind me. I'd hold my breath in an attempt to stifle any squeaks or whistles, and I'd sit on my hands to stop them from twitching too. It truly felt like my body was completely out of my control.

Eventually, I couldn't hold my tics in anymore and I whistled very loudly. A few people noticed and a couple of the teachers sent glares into the sea of students, thinking it was somebody misbehaving and trying to interrupt the assembly—this made me feel even more panicked because my worst fear as a student was being told off.

My neck was twitching more and more and my arms were moving too, so I knew I had to get out of there. I ducked down, slipped off my chair, and ran as quickly and quietly as I could down the edge of the hall until I reached the doors.

Once I escaped through the doors (which opened up to the nurse's office) my body exploded with jerks and noises so violently that I began to hit my chest and my head. My fist banged again and again on my chest, causing my collarbones to turn bright red underneath my blouse. I cried because I was alone and had no idea what was happening to me—it was terrifying!

It can be incredibly scary to experience these out-of-control tics when you don't know what's going on. It feels like your body is betraying you and that you're going to explode or hurt yourself accidentally. I felt like everybody would judge me and ask me why I was acting so weird, and I knew I couldn't give them an answer. I didn't know why!

I paced up and down the corridor, trying to let the tics pass, but it only carried on. I could still hear the assembly continuing, so I tried to make my vocal tics more quiet, but this only made them come out even louder.

I began shouting and screaming, and I even swore a few times involuntarily, which made me even more panicked and emotional. A few teachers walked by and stared at me as they passed, not understanding why I was behaving so "badly" and making so much noise. A few of them stared, which made me feel like I'd done something wrong—I felt my well-behaved student reputation crashing down. I was terrified of being judged when I couldn't control what was happening.

After about an hour of constant hitting, shouting, and whistling, my tics finally began to calm down and I managed to sit on the office sofa to calm my emotions down too. I was completely exhausted both physically and mentally.

After having my body out of control and moving constantly for so long, my muscles ached and my throat was already sore. The shouting made me lose my voice, and the hitting caused my knuckles and chest to become swollen and red. I knew it would later bruise, which worried me because I didn't know how to explain it to people. I didn't even know how to explain it to myself.

This was my first ever tic attack.

"The term 'tic attack' is often used to describe bouts of severe, continuous, non-suppressible and disabling tics which can last from a few minutes to several hours. They often include whole body writhing movements, muscle tensing and shaking."
  - Tourette's Action UK

I soon became very familiar with tic attacks, but this first one really caught me off guard. They are extremely exhausting and can last from a few minutes up to a few hours. My longest tic attack was over four hours long, and I've gained many injuries and even ended up in A&E (the emergency room in the UK) a few times.

When tic attacks happen, they can be very distressing and scary to experience (and also scary to witness). I never used to like having people near me in case they became worried, judged me, or worse… in case I accidentally hurt them.

I want to share a poem I wrote in early in my Tourette's journey which describes the feeling of tic attacks. I rarely share poetry (though I'm an avid writer) but I frequently use it to get all of my feelings out into my notes app.

Maybe some of you will relate to this feeling if you have tics yourself, or maybe you'll relate to some parts in a different way, as I know there are a lot of other reasons for feeling restricted or controlled in life.

I hate the feeling
    Of knowing what's about to come
    But being able to do nothing about it.
    I hate the feeling
    Of my own body betraying me,
    Never doing what I tell it to.

I feel the urge
    Like electricity in my spine,
    Bending me this way and that.
    Sounds come out of my mouth,
    And words
    I don't want so say, or even know.

I hate the feeling
    Of my muscles tearing apart,

My head swinging back too far
And my hand hitting my head
And my heart.

I hate not knowing
How long this will last.
Whether I'll come out unscathed
Or with a lasting scar?
All I do is sit and wait it out;
Letting my body become the puppet
To this force
I can never live without.

I don't want to move
This way and that;
Don't want to scream.
Or bruise my hands.
I want to sleep and stay in peace,
And live like the people around me.
But this is the life
My brain has chosen for me.

I sit and wait
for the attack to pass.
The worst moments leaving a
Memory that'll last.
I'm not sure what will happen next,
Nobody to predict or decide.
Forever it'll be just
Me and my brain,
Always just
Tourette's and me.

I know poetry isn't for everybody, so if you can't relate or connect with those words, then that's okay too! We all work in different ways, so you should never feel bad for preferring other methods or forms of creativity.

This poem spreads the message of how tic attacks are completely out of our control, and how in the moment, we are very aware of that fact. We can't decide what happens, and we rarely have any idea when attacks will happen or when they will stop. It's scary to experience and often quite lonely too, because nobody can truly understand what we're feeling in that moment unless they've been through it themselves.


This is why it's so important to seek out communities with similar conditions or struggles to yourself. The Tourette's community has done amazing things for me in terms of acceptance and feeling like I'm not alone—and I hope it can do that for you too! Please never feel afraid to reach out to your community on social media, or join groups in your area of the world to find people in similar situations. You never know how much it could help to hear other people's stories and be able to relate to them. Even if you're anxious or shy around new people, you can do it!

My community, my little corner of the huge online world, is such a friendly and nice space for people to hang out. I personally moderate a lot of the chats and comments to make it as safe a space as possible, and I have a team of moderators who manage my Discord server and social media to make sure complaints, negativity and hate are dealt with.

I know they'll be reading this, so I want to say a huge thank you to those friends for constantly keeping this community running and for making our corner of the internet feel like a safe place for all neurodivergent, queer, and disabled people all over the world. Everybody is welcome to come and make friends but I especially want to let disabled and neurodivergent people know that they're not alone, because I can personally relate to the experience of feeling like nobody understands or knows what I'm going through.

There are also countless neurodivergent Facebook groups, webinars, coffee mornings, in-person events in different countries, and charities (Tourette's Action provide support for people with TS in the UK, which I'll talk more about later) to find support in, so there is always a place you can look to find your people and find a home in the community.

∽

Not everybody with Tourette's experiences tic attacks, and not every tic attack is violent or loud. They can present differently in every person, and they can also present differently every time we have one. I've had many violent and hurtful tic attacks, some being purely physical and causing muscle exhaustion or injuries, but I've also had attacks that are entirely vocal, and some which don't come with any violent motor tics at all.

Tics can change severity over time, and they wax and wane continually. They may be more active for a few months and then become hardly noticeable for a while. However, this does not mean that the person's Tourette's has gone away. TS can't be cured, but there are many methods of managing and reducing tics in our day-to-day lives. Puberty is a common time for tics to become more severe, so my first tic attack and the timeline of my tics becoming more noticeable came right on cue, though I didn't know this at the time.

Tics are valid no matter their severity or whether they change day-to-day, and it's important we recognise that tics are a spectrum and look different in every case. You should never judge somebody's tics based on what you've seen another person's tics look like—everybody is different!

After my first tic attack, I knew that my tics weren't just brief twitches that would go away. I finally accepted that they were here, and they were becoming a problem. I couldn't concentrate in school, I was hiding from everybody, and these attacks caused severe physical pain.

This is when I captured the first recordings of my tics. I wasn't sure anybody would believe me when I eventually asked for help (and I am *notoriously* bad at describing the things I'm feeling, thanks alexithymia), therefore I documented each time an attack happened. I wrote diaries of my days, documented what my tics were like, and took videos whenever I had an attack so I could show the doctors what happens.


My elaborate plan to ask for help was "hindered" one day after a tic attack during the last lesson of my school day. I'd used my pass to leave yet another lesson, and was standing in the corridor to try and calm my tics down. Then, the bell rung.

It was the end of the day and my mum was waiting in the car park for me and my brother, but my tics were still really active. I didn't know what to do, as I knew I couldn't hold my tics in for the whole journey home, but I hadn't yet told my mum how much worse the tics had gotten. I was scared to tell anybody, even though my mum is a very understanding and accepting person.

I eventually made my way to the car and the tics continued to let themselves out. I sat in the back seat while my mum and my brother took the front seats. I kept seeing my mum sneak looks at me in the rear-view mirror, and I knew she'd noticed me moving and making weird noises. The car was completely silent for the entire journey. I don't think any of us knew what to say or how to react. It was completely new territory, and for my family it was probably a complete shock seeing me do these odd movements and sounds.

I felt so scared and self-conscious because I didn't know what was happening. It was one of those moments where I couldn't suppress the tics at all like when I usually tried to. My body was whistling, coughing, grunting, squeaking, meowing, and moving every limb in sudden jerks. It was pretty obvious in that moment that something was very wrong, so it came as a jarring surprise to my family and definitely took quite a while to get used to.

Please know that if you're at this stage of your Tourette's journey, that it will get better. The awkward stage is just that: a stage. It's just one of the many phases throughout the acceptance and adaptation period of getting a new diagnosis. It feels awkward to navigate at first, but it does get easier with time.

You'll find better ways of managing your tics, and the people around you will get used to them as they see them more and more. Being around understanding and open-minded people definitely makes this easier, but I like to believe everybody has a chance to adapt and be educated, so I always try to help people understand.

You may find it useful to print out or write down symptoms, or ways in which people can help you, and then give this to the people around you. Writing an email can feel easier than speaking in person, so do whatever works for you. Don't be afraid to ask for help so you can live more freely and get the adaptations and acceptance you need in order to move on with your life. You deserve support and equal opportunities, no matter your challenges or health conditions.

If you're reading and haven't experienced tics yourself, try to think about how you can help somebody going through this. Would you be accepting at first glance? Or would you instinctively back away at the unknown and assume the worst of somebody?

I know that before knew about Tourette's and developed it myself, I probably wouldn't have understood someone who was shouting or moving strangely in the street. I'd have probably tried not to stare, but maybe I wouldn't have offered a smile. I may have even felt afraid of the difference and strange behaviour.

Nowadays, I spend most of my time educating people on Tourette's and my other disabilities, trying to dispel this stigma, and taking steps to make the world feel like a slightly safer place for people who stand out. I want you to know that differences shouldn't be viewed as bad or scary, and they shouldn't be something we avoid. Disabilities don't make us any less, they just make us different.

If you see somebody in the street who is struggling with tics (maybe they're jerking their arms and legs or may shout words or make funny noises) please don't stare. But, if you catch their eye or glance at them, don't look away like you've been caught doing something wrong, because we're humans too and it shouldn't be treated like it's a crime to communicate with us!

That person in the street may have Tourette's syndrome, and they may be struggling or feeling embarrassed inside. I can think of so many occasions where I've been ticcing and I've felt like people are judging me, but I can also think of a few where people have smiled. If they've offered me a smile, it reassures me that I'm okay and that my tics didn't offend them.

I worry a lot about whether my tics might accidentally offend somebody or make them feel uncomfortable—even though I can't control them—so seeing people be friendly and "normal" towards me makes me feel like I'm welcome. It makes me feel accepted.

We should all try to be more open-minded and be friendly to whoever we can when we're out in the world, because you never know what is truly going on in somebody's life.

# EIGHT
# DIAGNOSIS

After months of my tics developing and becoming more disruptive and harmful, I finally managed to see a doctor.

We contacted my GP (general practitioner) who referred me to a paediatrician (a children's doctor) who then referred us to CAMHS—which in the UK is the Child and Adolescent Mental Health Service. Instead of seeing a neurologist, they referred me for counselling with CAMHS to help with anxiety, which they assumed was causing my tics.

However, after a few months we received a letter discharging me without assessment and without ever being seen. They passed my referral on to a mindfulness service, which I declined at the time out of pure frustration.

I was disappointed because I knew something was wrong, but none of the doctors would listen to me. I knew the tics didn't only happen when I was anxious, and that something different was happening to my body. The NHS waiting list to see a neurologist was over a year and a half long, and my GP said I'd have to wait at least eighteen months before getting seen. It would take even longer to actually get a diagnosis.

So, after these few referrals led nowhere and many months had passed by, my patience with my worsening tics was wearing thin. My mum eventually decided to get me a private referral instead of going through the NHS, which meant we had to pay for the appointments, but we'd get to see a neurologist within just a few weeks.

In early 2020, we paid for a private video call appointment with a specialist neurologist. After a few appointments with him (including assessments of my physical state, evaluating my tics, reviewing videos and symptoms, and talking about my history), I was finally given a diagnosis of Tourette's syndrome and also OCD (Obsessive Compulsive Disorder). These diagnoses are very common to have alongside each other and they both explained many things I'd dealt with from a young age.

Getting my TS diagnosis was a little scary because it confirmed that I had a lifelong neurological condition; I would never *not* have Tourette's after that moment. I knew my tics could change and get more severe or more mild over the months and years, but it took a while to get used to idea of having a new lifelong label.

The flip side of this, was the relief I felt after getting my diagnosis. It was confirmation of finally understanding what my body was doing. I could explain to people what was going on and explain my strange involuntary behaviours by using just one word: Tourette's.

This massively helped me in school, as people were quickly beginning to notice my worsening tics. Students stared at me and often assumed I was either coughing or being disruptive on purpose, which made my anxiety shoot through the roof.

I remember one day not long after my diagnosis, I stood in the corridor outside my English classroom after leaving a lesson where my tics had been really active.. My teacher then sent a misbehaving student out of room and he joined me in the empty corridor. I was shouting, whistling and hitting the wall without being able to stop—I was going into a tic attack.

I remember the student peeking his head around the corner and looking at me curiously as I ticced, then he asked me what I was doing. He sounded genuinely confused and curious, so I wanted to explain to him that they were tics.

"I have tics," I said to him, to which he replied with a confused raise of an eyebrow. He didn't know what tics were, and now I was out of explanations for him. I then said the word Tourette's, and he immediately nodded and understood what was going on.

This was the first time I remember telling somebody I had Tourette's, and the word felt clunky and strange coming from my mouth. I wasn't used to admitting I had this condition so it felt really weird at first! But despite the phrase feeling strange, I learned that having a name for my tics was really useful, it allowed me to quickly explain to people why I was randomly moving and making noises.

Since most people know a little bit about what Tourette's is. That singular word usually allows people to carry on with their days without judging me too much.

~

Although I've spoken about the development of my tics, you may be asking what Tourette's really is. Why does it happen, and what causes it? It's time again for a bit of science, but stick with me—I'm going to explain Tourette's in the most easily digestible way I can, while still giving you the facts.

Tourette's syndrome is a **neurological** condition (meaning it's caused by the brain) that causes involuntary movements and sounds called **tics**. These are categorised as **motor** and **vocal** tics, and can come in many different forms and severities.

Examples of motor tics could include: blinking, eye rolling, shoulder shrugging, jumping or touching objects and other people. And examples of vocal tics could include: grunting, throat clearing, whistling, coughing, tongue clicking, animal sounds, saying random words and phrases, repeating a sound, word, phrase or even swearing.

Not every person with TS has *all* of these tics, but you do need to have both motor and vocal tics (for over a year) to meet the criteria for Tourette's.

**Diagnostic criteria for Tourette syndrome include:**

- Multiple motor tics.
- One or more vocal tics.
- Tics which have lasted for more than one year (though they can wax and wane periodically).
- Tics starting before the age of 18.
- Tics that aren't caused by a drug or other medical condition.

Tourette's tics can start as early as the age of around four, but a diagnosis is only made after having tics for at least one year. Many people with TS go undiagnosed until their teen years because their tics aren't disruptive or noticeable enough to warrant investigation.

Studies have shown that about half of children with TS may not be diagnosed despite having had tics for many years. Tourette's is a spectrum, and as I've said earlier in the book, everybody's experience looks different!

TS is thought to be partly genetic, but a lot more research needs to be done to find out exactly which bit of our DNA causes

Tourette's to develop. Despite the condition being genetic and sometimes inherited from family, not all of us have tics for our entire lives. Usually, Tourette's will have an onset between the ages of 7-18 where the tics start and build up, however this is different for everybody. I didn't develop noticeable tics until the age of seven, and didn't get diagnosed until the age of fourteen when my tics hit their worst severity.

No matter what age you're diagnosed with Tourette's, or when your tics become more active, you are still valid! Nobody knows what you've been through better than you do, so please don't doubt yourself based on strangers' judgements or preconceptions.

~

Although Tourette's is what we first think of when we hear the word tics, TS isn't the only explanation for tics or the only condition which causes them.

In my case, Tourette's explained everything I'd been going through, and it gave me the clarity and validation I needed, but it's important to remember that tics don't always equal Tourette's syndrome.

There are other tic disorders which can explain tic symptoms; these can be diagnosed by a neurologist, so if you're worried about experiencing tics, please speak to your doctor.

This book is not a diagnostic tool and isn't intended for diagnostic use, so please remember that you should always consult a doctor before changing anything about how you treat, label, or manage symptoms. There are many causes for tics, so I advise you to do your own research and see a medical professional if you can.

There are a few different types of tic disorders, one being a persistent or **chronic** tic disorder, and another being a **provisional** tic disorder.


### Persistent (Chronic) Motor *or* Vocal Tic Disorder
To be diagnosed with a persistent tic disorder, a person must:

- Have one or more motor tics (for example, blinking or shrugging the shoulders) **or** vocal tics (for example, humming, clearing the throat, or yelling out a word or phrase), but *not* both.
- Have tics that occur many times a day nearly every day, or on and off for a period of more than a year.
- Tics start before the age of 18.
- Symptoms are not due to taking medicine or other drugs, or due to a medical condition which can cause tics.
- Not have been diagnosed with TS.


### Provisional Tic Disorder
To be diagnosed with a provisional tic disorder, a person must:

- Have one or more motor tics (for example, blinking or shrugging the shoulders) or vocal tics (for example, humming, clearing the throat, or yelling out a word or phrase).
- Tics present for no longer than 12 months in a row.
- Tics start before the age of 18.
- Symptoms are not due to taking medicine or other drugs, or due to a medical condition that can cause tics.
- Not have been diagnosed with TS, or a persistent motor or vocal tic disorder.

These are the medical diagnostic criteria for tic disorders, however people can also experience tics without having a tic disorder. Some medications such as ADHD medications or antipsychotics can cause tics as a side effect, and sometimes anxiety or stress can cause temporary bouts of tics. Children quite often have a tic or two (for example, blinking or scrunching their nose) at a young age, which then disappear as they grow older, so having one tic doesn't always mean they will develop into a disorder. It's best to monitor tic symptoms to see how long they stay and whether any more appear.

Tics are very common, and we shouldn't need to feel ashamed of ticcing in front of people. You are not strange, odd, or any less worthy than anybody else because you have tics, so please don't feel that you have to hide them in order to fit in.

If you're reading this and you don't have tics, please know that we can't control our tics: they're involuntary. We don't decide the sounds or the noises, and we can't control the volume, frequency or timing of our tics. We often don't even know what tics we're going to do until they come out—they surprise us too sometimes!

~

Before we move on, I'd like to teach you about the different types of tics, because although we know there are motor and vocal tics, there are actually many sub-categories of tics within these two umbrellas.

The first type is **echolalia** tics, which are the repetition of one's noises, words, or phrases. This tic is very common within the Tourette's community and often causes people with TS to have increased tics around other people with tics, because we trigger each other. Our tics repeat the things we hear, whether it's song lyrics, movie quotes, common words and phrases, or even the noises our pets make. One of my most common tics is a "meow" sound, which I can only assume I developed because of my cat, Jesse.

Similar to this is **palilalia**, which is the repetition of one's *own* words or phrases, which can often sound like stuttering as we repeat the same word over and over again.

Another type of repeating tic is **echopraxia**, which is similar to echolalia, but this time is the repetition of one's movements. This could mean our tics involuntarily copy people's jerking, facial twitching, waving, clapping, or even giving gestures like the middle finger or a peace sign.

The most commonly heard-of type of tic—though people don't often know the name for it—is **coprolalia**: the swearing tic. Tourette's is often referred to as "the swearing disorder" due to inaccurate portrayals in the media such as cartoon characters making rude comments and blaming it on "tics".

Although some people with Tourette's do say inappropriate words and phrases as tics (like me), this is only 10-15% of people with TS, meaning only a small percentage of us actually swear! This is a *huge* misconception of Tourette's, and it's one I always try to educate people on because our conditions are so often overlooked as funny or entertaining when this isn't the reality. Our tics can sometimes be funny (some of us do say words that may be entertaining) but more often than not, our tics are frustrating and disruptive.

Many people with Tourette's struggle to get jobs due to their tics becoming disabling, or employers not accepting the tics we may come out with. Sometimes people with tics can't drive because it isn't safe, or they can't go out alone because of the risk that somebody might misunderstand their tics and cause a confrontation.

I had to give up a lot of independence when my tics became very severe. I lost friends, missed countless lessons, fell behind in school, involuntarily ripped up exam papers after trying extremely hard to complete them, and I've never been able to get a "normal" job like my peers have.

Tourette's isn't a funny disorder that gives us an excuse to swear, it's an often very debilitating condition that causes us pain, misunderstandings, trouble finding and keeping jobs, difficulties concentrating… the list goes on.

But although people with Tourette's struggle to do many things because of our condition, we want you to know that we are just as capable and worthy as anybody else. We are smart and creative, and we know our condition's limits. We may not be able to do everything in the same way that people without Tourette's can, but we can adapt and do tasks in our own way so that our condition can co-occur. We can succeed in countless ways despite (and alongside) our tics, and we want you to know that we are people before we are our condition.

Tourette's affects our entire lives depending on the severity of our tics, but we don't let it control our lives. We have personalities, hobbies, and so many traits which aren't defined by our diagnosis. Please don't think of us as only a label or a joke between you and your friends. Remember that we are people.

The last type of tic I'd like to cover is **copropraxia**, which (like coprolalia) is a swearing tic. You may recognise the word's suffix **-praxia**, which indicates that this is a movement tic: copropraxia tics involve inappropriate movements and gestures. This may include giving the middle finger, making rude gestures or movements with genital references.

Like any other tic we do, we can't control these movements and we don't think of these before we do them. A person with

Tourette's doesn't look at somebody and *want* to flip them off—our bodies just do it without us ever even considering it!

It's so important for people to know this, because we are often judged for what our tics do when people assume we're the ones thinking of the tics. We're often made out to be horrible people behind the scenes because people assume Tourette's is an issue with having "no filter" but I can assure you this isn't true. I have never once wanted to give people the middle finger when I'm in public, and have never *actually* thought about swearing at the top of my voice in a supermarket—it just happens. My personality is nothing like what my tics portray.

This fact made it very uncomfortable to accept my tics at the beginning of my journey, because I feared people would view me differently. However, over time, I have gotten better at explaining misconceptions to people, and I no longer allow myself to feel looked down upon by individuals who don't understand my condition.

This isn't an extensive list of tic types, but here's a few more that you might like to research a little! There are -**graphia** tics which involve writing, and -**skepsi** tics which are mental tics that only happen in our thoughts; kind of like a word you just *can't* get out of your head. There are so many factors which can influence tics, and each person picks up tics from different places.

Now that you've learned a bit more about Tourette's, I hope you have some insight into what the condition entails and how it can be diagnosed. Tourette's is a lot to deal with and it's difficult to accept or come to terms with in itself, but it also often comes alongside other disorders too.

Up to 85 percent of people with TS have more struggles than just tics, due to co-occurring conditions such as OCD, ADHD, anxiety and autism being very common. I am also diagnosed with OCD, anxiety and autism, so I have experienced how these conditions all interact with one another.

Anxiety can cause tics to worsen with stress, and OCD triggers can make tics more active. Emotions often have a big impact on how active a person's tics are, despite Tourette's not being *caused* by stress.

In my experience, excitement, anxiety and frustration make my tics a lot more active. When I'm angry, my tics are usually more physical and may become dangerous or violent. When I'm excited, my tics are usually vocal and happen more frequently. But when I'm sad or suffering badly with depression, my tics often become very mild or can even go away completely on some days.

Everybody has different triggers for their tics, so it's best to explore your own body and find out what works for your own tics. Although I can give you my advice and personal experiences, every person responds slightly differently, so if you don't have Tourette's or tics yourself, then the best way to help and support other people with tics is to ask them what helps! Ask people what helps to reduce their tics, or if there's anything you can do to make things easier for them.

Some of my personal triggers for tics can be:

- stress or anxiety
- excitement
- people touching me (triggers motor tics)
- sugary foods or caffiene
- people repeating phrases (triggers vocal tics)
- seeing other people ticcing
- suppressing tics
- quiet spaces like libraries, churches & assemblies

And on the flip side, these are some things I've found that help my tics. Music helps me the most during a tic attack, but the other things on this list have massively reduced my tics over the years.

Some things which help my tics can be:

- listening to or playing music
- physical activity & sports (personally, I love yoga)
- concentrating on hobbies (for me, this includes reading, art & gaming)
- watching uplifting movies
- reading (especially before bed)
- reducing my sugar and caffeine intake
- keeping myself busy & distracted
- reducing time on screens & social media
- leaving school environments

We've not yet reached the point in my story of finishing school, but I'm going to cover how much this helped later on in the book. I know some of these ideas aren't accessible for everybody, but maybe something on this list can give you ideas for managing your tics. It's helpful to keep a diary or tracker for things that trigger your tics, or keep note of when tic attacks happen so you can spot any patterns or improvements.

# NINE
# STARTING SOCIAL MEDIA

Phew! That last chapter was a science heavy one, so I hope you've made it through and aren't completely overwhelmed. If you need to take a break, get up and do something which makes you feel good before coming back to the book with a fresh mind. If you're ready to carry on with my story, then read on and I'll take you through how I started posting on social media, detailing how content creation and advocacy became my hobby, and then my full-time job.

Shortly after my Tourette's diagnosis, I wanted to tell the people at school about my tics. They'd become so visible that I couldn't hide them any longer, therefore I knew I wanted to explain to people what was going on—but this is much easier said than done.

At school, I avoided lessons and suppressed my tics as often as I could, but this only provided a short-term solution as it caused a lot of tic attacks and frustration. After trying to explain to a few classmates in person, I decided that delivering information in person wasn't my speciality. At this point, I was incredibly shy, and my sentences were often interrupted by my vocal tics when I spoke to people. I needed to tell people what was happening and voice my needs in a way that was easily shared. This is when social media came into play!

I started by telling my friends on Snapchat and Instagram about what tics were and revealing that I had Tourette's. I posted a photo with the below caption and let my sixty-ish friends read it.

"So… I have Tourette's. Many people don't know because I hide it because it's embarrassing and even I don't yet fully understand it yet. I make strange facial expressions and make quick movements that sometimes make me look ridiculous or incredibly ugly which I am more than aware of, so please don't point this out.

I also make involuntary noises and say things I cannot control, for example swearing and telling people to shut up. I have no clue what comes out of my mouth until everyone else is hearing it too; these are tics and they are not aimed at anyone! It makes them worse and harder to deal with if people imitate or mock them or draw attention to them, so please keep that in mind.

Some tics can be funny (e.g one of my tics is "I'm a chicken nugget" like the vine) so it's okay to laugh along with me at the funny ones. But if I'm quite obviously stressed or in pain or uncomfortable, please ignore the tics and try to carry on as normal. Please don't draw attention to me as it makes it a lot more stressful.

I felt this was important to say because even though we're not in school at the minute, it's difficult to face people who don't understand what I'm going through. I deal with this every day and I have done for quite a while now, even though you probably haven't seen it outwardly.

Please be understanding and kind :)"

And that was how I told the people I went to school with! My first time telling my friends I had Tourette's was via this exact message which I uploaded just before going back to school (during the first Covid 19 lockdown) to give allow a few weeks for the information to sink in.

I highly recommend using a online post, text message or writing a paragraph with educative facts as a way to explain to people what's going on. It's helpful to include your own preferences for how you'd like people to react and help you feel comfortable. Feel free to use mine as a template if you're struggling! Writing definitely helped me feel more comfortable and start educating people even with my first posts being short and sweet. I now have much more knowledge and experience when people ask me about tics, but this was a really important first step.

My first *public* post about my tics was actually a short while before my diagnosis. I posted a video on TikTok of me singing along to music, and added text on the screen saying "When my tics decide to swear when somebody comes into my room" before pulling a horrified face. A few of my friends found this funny and asked me about my tics in the comments, so it opened up an opportunity to explain how frustrating my tics were. It felt good finally to talk about it, so I continued posting.

I looked very different back then; I didn't wear any colourful clothing at all, I always styled my hair in front of my face to hide my cheeks, and I spoke very quietly and softly. Even my tics seemed more awkward back then because I wasn't as confident about letting them out!

I had *zero* stage presence in front of a camera like I do now, so back then my videos felt so awkward! These days, I'm pretty confident when recording content and my videos are more like a casual chat—but back then, I was highly masked with not much personality. This really shows the effects of masking and how neurodivergent people are often afraid to be themselves because they fear being judged.

After making a few more videos, I decided to record a talking video using my own voice. I filmed a short Q+A video on TikTok for Tourette's awareness month, which is from the 15th May to the 15th June every year. This was my first time celebrating Tourette's awareness month after receiving my diagnosis, so I took it as an opportunity to share my story and start educating people.

This video received hundreds of views, which was a lot more than my usual two hundred followers at the time. This made me happy because I wanted more people to learn about Tourette's, I wanted to help spread the message of what it really looked like. I researched for hours, finding out all the statistics and facts for Tourette's, and it quickly became a huge interest of mine.

I'd now consider neurology and TS to be a special interest of mine since learning about special interests during my autism diagnosis. The brain and the way it works have interested me, so I viewed my Tourette's diagnosis as a learning opportunity and this made it a lot easier to accept and deal with.

I continued making videos throughout Tourette's awareness month, and some of them reached a thousand views, which seemed like so many back then! Soon after, I posted my first ever viral video titled "Things I can't do because of my Tourette's" where I spoke about the day-to-day things that my Tourette's made it difficult to do—for example going to the cinema or playing hide and seek.

Within twenty-four hours, this video hit hundreds of thousands of views, and eventually hit one million. I couldn't believe it! I'd never reached or even imagined this many people before; the thought of one million people seeing my face made me a bit nervous. I spent the whole day figuring out how to feel about it, and replying to the thousands of comments.

Some of these comments were mean, and showed that some people didn't understand why I was making funny noises despite the title of the video stating my condition. However, many of the comments *were* genuine people who were curious to learn more. They didn't know what Tourette's was and the new information fascinated them! I replied to these comments and posted more videos answering different questions about my tics. I also started posting challenges after seeing a few other people try to hold an egg with their tics, or try to say the alphabet and see how their tics responded.

I quickly learned that people on the internet love entertainment, and since my tics often say a lot of funny words, this was the perfect combination for making people laugh. People loved to watch as I tried and failed to complete tasks with my tics interrupting, and they loved to watch baking attempts where my tics jerked and threw eggs. It was easy-to-make content that millions of people happily watched.

This was fun at first! I loved talking about my tics, and I felt like I was making a difference as I educated so many people on Tourette's in videos where I talked about my experiences and listed facts. I loved answering people's questions when they said they didn't know what TS was or what it involved. I found that I really, really loved educating.

Posting about my tics ignited a passion for advocacy and content creation. I loved researching, recording videos, talking about Tourette's, editing videos, getting cool cameras shots, writing descriptions, and uploading YouTube videos.

I fell in love with the whole process, and this spurred me forward to keep uploading nearly every day on TikTok for years, and nearly every week on my YouTube channel. I didn't earn a penny from the first two to three years of my creator journey, which sometimes surprises people to hear! I spent hours and hours editing, researching, putting videos together, filming and replying to comments... and I never earned any money from those daily TikTok videos! I did it because I loved meeting people and teaching them about my condition. I loved finding a space and a community where I wasn't afraid to show my tics. It was a place where I didn't have to hide.

I also found countless people who were grateful for me sharing my story because they were in similar positions, and they could relate to my content. This made me feel so warm inside. I loved hearing people's stories and reading through hundreds of messages describing how people felt seen and understood—it made me feel like all the effort I'd put it really was making a difference. Every minute was worth it.

My content has definitely changed over the years, reshaping itself as I grew older and documented finishing school, and then college. You can see how I change both physically and mentally if you scroll through my accounts, and I also become so much more knowledgeable about my conditions and what I've been through.

I don't post many challenge videos anymore, and I try to focus on more educative content because I've realised that although people react well to tic videos (views are usually higher when I post my funnier tics), this isn't the *only* thing I want people to see about my condition. I want to educate people on the reality of Tourette's and part of this was accepting that only posting funny compilations of my tics doesn't help deconstruct the misconceptions behind Tourette's or coprolalia, because it leaves out an entire plethora of struggles and daily realities of living with tics.

It's so important to share the facts and the real stories behind what TS affects in our lives, and yes, this does include funny tics too! We sometimes say funny things if our tics are verbal (verbal tics are words and phrases, whereas the term vocal covers any type of noise), and 10-15% of us also have swearing tics. So, this is still an important thing to show if we want to educate on the complete picture of TS.

It's very easy to lose sight of what's helpful when the algorithm promotes funny and entertaining content instead of the videos that truly matter or make a difference. When I was younger and made videos, I just wanted to make people happy and ensure that they enjoyed my content, so I mainly posted my funniest tics.

This is something I've recently tried to reshape after taking a big break from posting any videos of my tics. I think it's important for us people with Tourette's to show our symptoms *within* our daily lives, but also show ourselves! We should include our hobbies, and things that help our tics, as well as the things that don't. I love to make art and music, so I post a lot about the things I'm doing creatively as well as making vlogs of fun trips, detailing how my conditions affect what I'm doing.

My advice to anybody wanting to share their tics or start posting online, is to do so in a way that doesn't promote only the funny side, because you deserve to be seen for more than just your tics' jokes. You deserve to be treated with respect.

If you feel comfortable, it's often helpful to show the hard, sad and difficult sides of living with Tourette's too. It's important to show the things we struggle with behind the scenes and educate on the tics people don't immediately think of, such as internal motor tics like breathing or clenching our stomach muscles.

The internet can be a huge and intimidating space, so make sure to only share what you feel comfortable with, but know that any educative posts you do share are so valuable to our disabled community.

# TEN
# ARE YOU THERE?

Overlapping with my Tourette's journey, I developed another set of symptoms which didn't fit with my TS diagnosis.

It began in 2019, when I first started to experience fainting, drop attacks and strange episodes where my limbs would stop working. At this stage in life (the year before my Tourette's diagnosis) I instinctively hid what I was going through, therefore I didn't immediately tell anybody about these new symptoms. I spent most of my school days alone in corridors or hiding in the toilets, therefore I often had these unconscious episodes while nobody was there. I sometimes didn't realise I'd even had an episode if my brain was still "fuzzy" afterwards.

To younger me, hiding my health issues felt like the only option; I felt so embarrassed and confused. I instinctively masked any new struggles due to my previous battles with mental health, so when these new physical symptoms started, my instinct was to shut off from people. I wanted to hide everything that was different or "weird" which in hindsight, was probably to avoid being bullied again. During a lot of secondary school, all I strived to do was blend in and disappear into the crowd so that I could live my life in peace… but alas, life doesn't always let you do that!

I began having absence seizures, which are episodes where the person looks like they're staring into space or "freeze" for a minute or two. Usually mine involve some twitching of my face or eye-rolling, and I'll feel very "out of it" or drowsy both before and afterwards. These usually last between ten seconds to a couple minutes, however my friends have said that some episodes lasted over twenty minutes or more without fully coming around in between each seizure: these are called seizure clusters.

When these episodes began, I didn't understand what was happening at all. Since I didn't know what seizures looked or felt like back then, I had no idea that my episodes were actually non-epileptic seizures for quite some time.


Another type of episode I experienced was sleep attacks. I'd be sitting in class when suddenly I'd feel really out of it, and people's words would blur together. I couldn't hear the teacher properly, and my vision went all fuzzy as my eyes unfocused. My arms started to feel like bricks; I couldn't lift them off the table even if I tried with all my concentration, so I'd lay my head on my desk and shortly afterwards, pass out.

This began happening more and more, until it became every few weeks, then every week, and then every day. I'd feel symptoms coming on and so I'd set my head on the table and prepare myself. The next thing I'd remember was waking up and trying to lift my head despite it feeling like the heaviest thing in the world. Sometimes my friends reported that I twitched or shook slightly in my "sleep" which made me even more confused as to what was happening. Why was I losing consciousness so much?

When people couldn't get my attention during these episodes, teachers sometimes became frustrated thinking I wasn't paying attention and that I was just staring into space or sleeping on my desk, when in reality my head felt so fuzzy. I couldn't hear them properly or respond and I didn't understand what was going on or what people were saying during these episodes. It was extremely confusing to go through as a student, especially when nobody around me knew what seizures were or what the signs could look like. This is why it's so important to raise awareness for seizure first aid, so that if somebody experiences a seizure episode in school or in public, people know how to help and care for them until they come around, or until help gets there.

One of my first episodes was in 2019. I was in year nine, and I remember being in a music lesson at school. I started to feel dizzy and strange, so I asked to step outside. I took my water with me and tried to deep-breathe away the odd, uncomfortable feeling. I started to feel like I wasn't really there; my vision blurred and my head felt like it was spinning. My arms had no strength in them, and my knees buckled as I paced the corridor.

I remember sliding my back down the wall and sitting propped up in the bright yellow corridor of the music department. I sat waiting for the feeling to pass, feeling terrified that something bad was going to happen because I'd never felt this woozy before. In this moment, I set my phone up to record so that I could see what happened while I was unconscious and show it to somebody later on if I needed to. I lay my head back against the wall behind me and slowly started to fall unconscious. I only know what happened after this due to rewatching the video footage, so I'm really glad I decided to set up my phone!

My eyes unfocused, becoming vacant with no real expression. My arms dropped along with my whole body, then after a few minutes, my face and jaw began to convulse (this is where your muscles twitch or shake repeatedly). I now know this episode to be a partial seizure, which is in between an absence seizure and a full-body convulsive seizure. For me, they usually look similar absence seizures (staring into space) but these also come along with some mild convulsions.

Partial seizures feel really strange to experience because I often slip in and out of consciousness as the seizure is happening, resulting in a few foggy memories of being awake during these. It's never nice to remember a seizure because my brain feels incredibly cloudy. I'm confused and my body usually hurts if I'm tensed or convulsing repetitively.

After this particular seizure finished and I was responsive again, I felt quite emotional. Seizures often leave you completely drained. It felt like I could nap for a entire day, but I knew I had to go back to class... so I did. I told my friend I hadn't felt well and tried to rest as much as I could in between tasks, but I eventually went to the school nurse so I could sit in a quiet room and properly have some time out.

This is the first seizure I have actual documentation of, but I slowly began recording a lot more of my seizures either by writing down details and timings, or by filming them so I could see what happening while I wasn't aware.

I eventually worked up to telling my mum what was happening, and we had a long chat about my symptoms and what was going on, eventually deciding that contacting the doctor was the best idea. When we finally got an appointment with my GP, he asked us to collect evidence (video footage) of my seizures, therefore all the videos I'd already taken were incredibly useful—I'd instinctively recorded my episodes already!

It took months of waiting to finally get an appointment and my symptoms worsened over the time it took to finally get seen. My seizures became more frequent and I was fainting at school any time I stood up too quickly or if had to stand for long periods. I knew something in my body wasn't right, and the new symptoms felt so different from any tic or experience I'd had with my anxiety or Tourette's. My days were blending together with the episodes and foggy consciousness, so I just focused on getting through the school day without having to be sent home early to rest.

This struggle was then interrupted by a time we'll all never forget... Covid 19.

# ELEVEN
## COVID 19

The world seemed to come to a complete standstill in 2020, as this never-before-heard-of pandemic spread across the world. A mysterious virus was causing illness and an increasing amount of recorded deaths. I remember this whole situation feeling like a fever dream at the time; I couldn't believe what I was hearing or seeing on the news. It seemed like the script of an action film where the end of the world is coming and the population soon turns against one another. We were all terrified at first!

The world declined into a situation where our governments didn't know what to do, since our generation had never experienced a pandemic like this before. The world felt full of fear, and the outcome of the next few months was completely unknown.

The first time we went into lockdown in the UK, I didn't believe it would really happen. I was struggling a lot at school, so my mind was preoccupied with my symptoms and managing my tics. But suddenly, the Prime Minister was talking about shutting the country down and establishing isolation rules, closing schools, having a curfew and only being advised to go out for a ten-minute daily walk. It was so strange—I remember sitting in the living room with my family and watching the announcements on the TV, feeling like we were in *The Purge*!

In the UK, all of our schools closed—this was originally for two weeks, however closures ended up lasting for months. This caused immense disruption with our education as online learning wasn't set up until later that year, so I remember all of my friends doing little to no school work for about two or three months.

We sat at home, waiting for the next weekly announcement and spending our time on social media, scrolling TikTok and watching video after video. This excited me at the time because I was just beginning to post about my tics online, therefore I used my newfound free-time to make more videos talking about my recent diagnosis of Tourette's. I also found another reason to enjoy the isolation of lockdown: I could hide my tics.

I didn't have to go to school in person any more, therefore I didn't have to suppress my tics every single day or spend my time in corridors trying to compose myself. I didn't have anybody asking questions or wondering why I was making noises. I didn't have to worry about hiding anything!

While Covid caused a lot of tragedy in the world and lockdown interrupted the economy of the country, the break from socialising actually served as a barrier between me and other people while I figured out how to deal with my tics. I could accept, understand and learn to live with my tics without the views or questions of anybody else, and I think this is one reason I'm now so confident in talking about my tics. Adapting to a new diagnosis is always a really difficult adjustment to go through, but this did allow me to process everything at my own pace.

I'm definitely privileged in the sense that I could stay home and didn't have to work like so many of the nurses and doctors saving lives every day. I was a teenager who could sit in the house and safely wait out the pandemic therefore, although

Covid was scary and the threat of getting sick was still there, I never truly saw the horrific reality a lot of first responders saw during this time. I want to acknowledge everybody who struggled and risked themselves during this time to help others. You all helped to keep our world running during this weird and very unsettling time.

~

I began to struggle with my OCD a lot more during lockdown, spurred on by the real fears of contamination. I suffer with contamination OCD, meaning I am in constant hyper-vigilance about germs, washing my hands, or not touching anything in public such as door handles and touchscreens. It makes life difficult on harder days, but I'm gradually getting better at rationalising these thoughts and challenging compulsions.

However, during the start of Covid, these things terrified everybody. My irrational fears of touching people, breathing the same air as people, washing any germs off my hands and so on... had actually become real. It wasn't my OCD making me afraid any more, because everybody in the world was *also* afraid of contamination. The threat was real this time.

This made my OCD incredibly difficult to cope with. My thoughts spiralled quicker than ever, and I was afraid to even step out of my house. I couldn't go into my bathroom, I struggled to go into my kitchen and I wouldn't let anybody near any of my food. I also struggled to touch or stand close to anybody— even my own family.

Whilst my thoughts spiralled with contamination fears, this irrational thinking also affected other aspects of my life. I became very "picky" with what I could eat, only choosing safe textures which didn't make me feel uncomfortable. I ate only toaster waffles for weeks of my life during those months, and that isn't over-exaggerating! This is a genuine struggle a lot of autistic people and children go through, and in some cases can lead to an eating disorder called ARFID.

A lot of foods didn't feel "safe" to put into my body, and I frequently broke down over textures of food, clothing, or things I touched. I struggled to dress myself and wear any clothing because it felt wrong on my body. Even the sound of certain words distressed me because they didn't sound *right* when being said. I thought this was all caused by OCD at the time, but I now know that autism exacerbated this for me, despite having had no idea I was actually autistic at the time.

Lockdown was a very surreal time and apart from the struggles I've mentioned, I mostly don't remember much of it. A lot of you can probably relate when I say those months are a black hole in our memories. My next memorable moment picks up when I finally went back to school, and I had to take a Covid test on my first day back.

# TWELVE
# THE COVID TEST

Not to sound dramatic, but one Covid test pretty much changed my life. My entire world shifted and start morphing into what it is now, after my first day back at secondary school during the pandemic.

After months of lockdown, we were finally told we could come back to school. And while this was good because we could start learning again, it was also terrifying because it meant I had to see people in person.

My tics had become *even* more severe during our time away from school. They'd sent me to A&E multiple times for tic attacks, which left my knuckles bruised and swollen. I'd developed a lot more swearing tics, different phrases, and even entire sentences as vocal tics. I was shouting, kicking, and falling down, my tics bucking my knees when walking. My tics were very severe in 2020 and 2021, and the stress of the pandemic definitely made them a lot worse.

Despite posting more on social media (and gaining over 400,000 followers) some people at my school still didn't know I had Tourette's. My tics changed a lot during the months of lock-down, so the loud and disruptive involuntary outbursts came as a real shock to my classmates and teachers when I went back to school.

My mum set up meetings with my teachers to put a care plan in place for me, and we had to explain to all the staff why I was swearing and hitting myself. I probably looked and acted like a completely different person. I'd gone from the introverted, shy girl who leaves lessons crying (but quietly works hard and gets good grades), to a girl who shouts obscenities and punches walls involuntarily.

I was so embarrassed at first; I couldn't fathom seeing the people I'd grown up with and letting them witness what my life had turned into. They gave me strange looks and everybody laughed at any jokes or any swear words my tics said. I suddenly became the jokester in classes, even though all I wanted to do was sit quietly, blend in and work hard.


On the first day back, my mum came in with me because I was so nervous that my tics became really active. I couldn't stop moving and jerking my body, and my tics shouted and whistled uncontrollably.

In the school hall, everybody stood in lines preparing to have their Covid tests done. I felt exposed and embarrassed, so my teacher led my mum and I to a separate testing room. My tics were increasing, and since I'd never taken a Covid test before, they quickly become extremely active with the nerves. Building up and up and up, I reached a tic-attack-level of tics.

When the teachers gave us the Covid test, they left us alone for five minutes so we could get the test done without the pres-sure of anybody watching me (this was a very helpful adapta-tion). After about two minutes of trying to get the swab anywhere near my face, my mum and I were rolling around with laughter—my tics just *wouldn't* let it happen. I was pulling funny faces involuntarily, karate chopping the swab stick, leaning backwards as far as my body could... it was a nightmare!

But we definitely found humour in this tricky situation, and as we continued trying, it became absolutely comical. My mum turned to me and said through her laughter, "You should be filming this, it's hilarious," and I laughed, thinking she was joking. She turned back to me and suggested that it would be a good part of Tourette's for people to see, as they probably don't realise how tricky living with tics can be. I wholeheartedly agreed with her.

People don't usually consider how having Tourette's could affect something as simple as taking a Covid test, so in that moment I knew I wanted to document my experiences and show the world what life can look like with my condition. I wanted to show people how day-to-day tasks can be incredibly tricky when you have tics, even when they seem easy to everybody else.

We set up my phone to record and carried on trying to get the test done. It took around fifteen minutes (though I only filmed just over a minute) to actually get the swab in my nose, and I still jerked away once it was in my nose. This was quite painful—it's not very nice having a stick up your nose and then suddenly jerking around!

Although this may surprise many of you who saw that video, we did actually get the test done! The teachers sent me to class when the negative line showed up, so I took a deep breath, said goodbye to my mum, and I officially returned to school.

My first day was absolute chaos. I felt really embarrassed about my tics because there was absolutely no way of hiding them;

they were too severe. My Tourette's was out—loud and proud—for the entire class to see and hear.

People did ask questions; I had to explain myself over and over again and I quickly knew the Tourette's definition off by heart. I found I quite liked telling people the facts because I knew many statistics from the research I did for my more educational videos. I enjoyed educating people, however it *was* a lot more difficult in person.

Kids in British secondary school aren't always nice—correction, they're often incredibly mean and don't wish to change—so, although I spent much of the day explaining my Tourette's, how I developed it, why I said weird things, whether I could control it, and so on… negative rumours still started to spread.

When I got home on first day of school, I was *exhausted*! My whole body ached from moving constantly, especially my neck from all the sudden neck jerks. I fell straight into bed, something that would become a daily occurrence from then on.

After taking a nap, I went back to look at the Covid test footage I'd filmed and it was quite amusing. Of course, it showed the struggle, but it was also entertaining! This humour is the side of Tourette's that was easier to show to people because it makes them laugh and everybody likes to be entertained. Focusing on this positive aspect of my tics eased the awkward atmosphere around my condition. It made me see something good that could come out of developing it.

I edited the video and later that day, posted it to TikTok. It had "only" two thousand views before I went to bed—lower than my average at the time—therefore I assumed it wouldn't do well at all. I went to bed and pushed it to the back of my thoughts.

In the morning, I checked my phone and saw that I had a message from Buzzfeed on Instagram! Buzzfeed?! I knew I had quite a lot of followers for a teenager, but getting contacted by such an enormous company seemed unbelievable. I checked the message and they'd sent me a screenshot of my video with two million views, saying they'd like to feature it and help share my story.

I scrambled to the TikTok app, and—low and behold—my video of the Covid test had over seventeen *million* views. My jaw dropped. I didn't know what to think!

I nervously told my mum, who completely freaked out because she was also in the video. My mum doesn't really like being on camera, but she doesn't mind if I make video alone. The amount of views came as a real shock to her, and we were both nervous about receiving hate comments because we knew the internet wasn't always a safe place.


That morning, I logged onto my school lesson as usual (we still had some of them online) and I told my form teacher about the video . I checked the views after my first lesson and it climbed to over twenty-five million. As a few days passed, it got to thirty, then forty, fifty... and so on. My followers jumped from four hundred thousand to one million in only two days, which was completely surreal. I celebrated by watching a follower counter with my dad and filming my reaction—I felt so fulfilled!

But of course, the viral video did result in a lot more hate. My videos were consistently reaching over a million views, so I discovered a new sense of pressure to post. People were critiquing my every move, and I felt scared to post videos in case people didn't like them, or in case I accidentally represented Tourette's wrongly. I feel like I had a huge role to play, and like the weight of it fell all on my shoulders.


I remember a few videos after the Covid test, I posted a TikTok where my tics were particularly active. My coprolalia (the swearing tics) were acting up, and my tics said a few rhyming phrases which wouldn't be okay to say voluntarily. I included these in the video with a comment telling people that this was involuntary, and that Tourette's can cause inappropriate words and phrases to become tics. I told people not to say the words if they can control it, because they would be offensive.

The internet jumped onto this quicker than I could register what was happening. The comments flooded with people telling me I was racist, a bad person, and much worse—it made me so upset. I'd wanted to show the real side of Tourette's and be honest about *everything* the condition entails. I didn't want to only show the funny side, or the side that people liked because that just wasn't accurate.

Tourette's can cause tics that aren't nice, tics which don't conform with social norms, and tics which may be uncomfortable to hear—but we can't control it. We don't think of our tics before we say them and we don't choose what to tic, or when to tic it.

Being out in public can be really scary for somebody with coprolalia, because we never know when our tics will say something that could get us in trouble or something which might offend somebody. If we tic in the wrong scenario, it could put us in danger.

I didn't go out by myself for a very long time after my tics got worse. I was terrified of being judged or overheard by someone who might start a fight. I constantly had a fear of being beaten up, and I was terrified of offending people in public and not having a chance to explain why I was saying or doing those things.

People often stare at me in public, but they rarely ask what's going on or give me any chance to explain what Tourette's is. They scowl or look at me disapprovingly before walking off or quickly looking away. I'm grateful that I haven't had many confrontations, but it's also really disheartening when I don't have a chance to explain why my body moves like this, or why I say things I can't control. It makes me sad when people perceive my tics as me being nasty, violent, or badly behaved simply because they don't know it's involuntary.

This is why spreading awareness for Tourette's is so important, and why I advocate for every side of the condition. I try to share the funny parts, the hurtful parts, the painful parts, the offensive tics, the invisible tics, and everything that comes with having TS. It isn't all fun and games, though that's what the media usually shows. TS affects hundreds of thousands of people's lives, and it often prevents us from doing the things we love.

If you're reading this and you don't have tics, please try to be more open-minded about people who are different. Offer them smiles in public, ask them politely if you have a question when you're curious, and respect their answer whether they say yes or no. Help educate people who may pre-judge Tourette's, and maybe even tell them some facts you learned in this book!

My primary goal of posting online has always been to make society a little safer for people like me, and to help make Tourette's more well-known and better understood. I want to increase the chance of somebody understanding when they see somebody in public who's ticcing, because it can make the difference between us feeling ashamed of our tics, and feeling accepted by a smiling stranger.

If you have Tourette's and you've experienced inappropriate tics, or you've been judged for something your tics have said, then you are not alone. There is an entire community of people out there who have experienced similar things, and I can promise you that your tics are *not* your fault. If you can't help what tic comes out, then you shouldn't have to feel bad or embarrassed about the tic!

Awareness and sensitivity around coprolalia tics is so important, because we need to find a balance where everybody is comfortable. People have a right to feel hurt or offended when hearing slurs, but people with Tourette's also have a right to live freely despite their involuntary condition. The general public shouldn't use offensive language or slurs, but people also need to understand that Tourette's isn't controllable. We need people to understand that we don't *want* to tic hurtful things. We don't want to tic negative phrases, slurs, or be physically violent. Tics are involuntary, and they don't represent who we are underneath.

~

After my video went viral, everybody in my school knew about my tics. The video reached over ninety-million views and featured on nearly every social media platform and even in the news. People started to recognise me when out shopping, which was a bizarre experience! It's nice to meet people in real life (most of you have been so kind), but it was definitely a weird feeling for strangers to know my name and ask to take a photo with me.

Every teacher at my school saw the video too, and most of the students from other years recognised me in the corridors when walking to lessons. They soon gave me the nickname "TikTok girl" which people shouted down the corridor if they saw me. I wasn't so sure how to feel about this—it was frustrating whenever I'd leave a lesson feeling very anxious or ticcing badly and somebody would stop me in the corridor to ask me if I was "that girl from the TikTok video" while I tried to fend off my incoming panic attack.

I'm not afraid to admit that I really struggled. I wanted to disappear again, so that I could deal with everything on my own and in private, especially since my health was worsening again. The longer I was at school for, the more my stress increased... and if you know anything about FND, then you'll know that stress is our worst enemy.

# THIRTEEN
## EXAM SEASON

When my tics reached their worst and my videos were mega-viral, I was in year ten of secondary school (age 14). This meant I had just started my GCSEs. The focus on grades became more important, and we were told to revise every day. Lockdown had interrupted our studies for a while, but after returning to school, the exam pressure came straight back—this time in the form of classwork-based assessments.

This immense amount of stress soon triggered my other symptoms to worsen. My fainting and seizure episodes continued, but they progressively worsened into 2020.

I developed new symptoms where my feet curled inwards and locked, leaving them completely rigid. I struggled to walk when this happened, so I used crutches to get around my school. My legs often lost their strength and became floppy after I had seizures, and my arms felt too heavy to move, which could last for up to an hour.

I spent an increasing amount of time at the nurse's office, and my mum frequently picked me up from school early. If I'd had a seizure and I was exhausted, or a body part stopped working temporarily, then my mum would come and take me home to rest.

After a particularly nasty seizure one night at home, I woke up to find my legs completely paralysed. I couldn't move a muscle anywhere from the waist down, which was more than I'd ever experienced before—I couldn't even shift my weight from side to side.

I remember calling my mum and telling her I couldn't move my legs. We couldn't figure out what was happening, so she tried to help me stand while using my crutches for balance. Though this usually worked when my legs locked up, this time I flopped straight to the floor—I couldn't bear any weight on them. Around this time, my mum called the doctor and we scheduled an appointment to start finding answers, but it would *still* be months before I even was seen.

That year, I went to school using crutches on more days than not. I always had some sort of brace on to try to hold my bent and rigid limbs into place and reduce pain, or to give my partially paralysed legs some strength. I left most of my lessons early to give me more time to get to the next classroom and I always brought a friend to make sure I got there safely. I quickly fell behind in classes and my tics were interrupting more than ever.

When I tried to suppress my tics, they'd become so active afterwards that I'd go straight into a tic attack. I remember having tic attacks outside nearly every one of my classrooms. I'd let most of my tics out at break time, therefore my friends saw the progression of my tics at their worst. My best friend at the time would hold my hands when the tics became violent, trying to help by putting soft things in between my knuckles and the wall, or placing a padded coat on the table. She'd laugh along if my tics said funny words and we joked when I said phrases about chickens (one of my most common tics at the time).

I had some pretty nasty injuries in years ten and eleven

because my tics would hit the table repeatedly, causing my knuckles to turn purple and blue. I used more ice packs than I can count, going back to the nurse for one every time I had a tic attack. The nurse frequently put a sling on me after my arms paralysed during the day because this helped keep the circulation flowing instead of the arm just dangling by my side.

My health quickly became more debilitating as these physical symptoms became out of control. My tics controlled my social life significantly, but my seizures and other FND symptoms completely flipped my life upside down.

I remember sitting in class one day when I felt a seizure aura coming on. I always called this my "fuzzy feeling" because I didn't know much about seizures at the time. I went to sit in a quiet room in the learning support department, and after sitting for a while, I fell to the side and my memory blacked out. I have a few snippets of memory of feeling the floor on my face and twitching, but I couldn't remember anything when I first woke up. I'd had my first full tonic-clonic seizure at school… in front of a teacher.

For those of you who don't know, a **tonic clonic** seizure (sometimes called a grand-mal seizure) is when the person loses consciousness and may fall. The **tonic** part of the seizure involves muscles contractions which can force air out of the lungs and cause gasping or gurgling sounds, even if the person isn't aware of their surroundings. The person may drool or accidentally bite their tongue or cheek in a severe seizure. In some cases, breathing can be affected, which could make the person's face turn bluish or gray due to lack of oxygen.

My seizures are non-epileptic, meaning I don't have epilepsy. Epileptic seizures can be extremely dangerous if left untreated and can even cause death, whereas a non-epileptic seizure isn't "inherently dangerous" because they don't cause direct damage to the brain. However, non-epileptic seizures can still be dangerous if the person falls and hits their head, or if they can't breathe during the seizure, so it's still necessary to monitor these carefully.

**NEAD** (non-epileptic attack disorder) is a common diagnosis to be given alongside the umbrella term of FND. Other names sometimes used for non-epileptic seizures are "Dissociative seizures" or "Psychogenic Non-Epileptic Seizures" also known as **PNES**. The psychogenic part of this name often throws people off, as they think this means the seizures aren't real or that they're "just in our heads", but this term actually refers to one cause of seizures being linked with psychology.

For many cases of FND, symptoms can be caused by trauma, stress, prolonged anxiety or other psychological causes. In these cases, the seizures are somewhat like the brain's way of shutting off when everything becomes too much. Our brains get overloaded (this can be subconscious) and the signals stop connecting properly, leaving our bodies in a state of dysfunction. However, not all FND cases follow this timeline, therefore the psychogenic label is thankfully being used less and less as more research is done on the condition.

I believe chronic stress and being undiagnosed autistic to be part of my FND onset as it developed during such a traumatic point in my life, however some FND patients don't have *any* previous mental health struggles and may develop symptoms after a head injury, a physical injury, illness or even at random.

∼

I don't remember when my very first seizure was, but my first seizure in school has always stuck in my memory. My cheek hurt from rubbing against the scratchy carpet, and I felt so fuzzy and confused when I came out of it. I felt embarrassed that my teacher saw me in such a vulnerable state, even though she already knew I had these episodes from reading my care-plan.

We still didn't have any medical answers, so I didn't yet have a diagnosis to confirm what caused these episodes, but we quickly knew they were seizures. I recorded the details of episodes in my notes app and continued to take notes every time I had seizures or new symptoms for the next few months.

I'd like to share some of these daily entries to show you how often FND can affect somebody's life, and how much we truly go through every single day. I updated this list for a good year and a half before I lost count, but in just that period, I noted over four hundred seizures.

**Sunday 18/04/21**

- absence seizures all day
- 6 minute partial seizure (8pm, felt weird/slow)
- seizure (9pm)

**Tuesday 20/04/21**

- seizure when waking up (7.10am)
- absence with teacher (10am)
- faint (lasted 5 mins, bit my tongue during)
- hands locked up (11.45am)
- absence into full seizure (21.20pm)

**Wednesday 21/04/21**

- hands paralysed all day (arms periodically paralysed too - no movement at all)
- absence seizures all day

- passed out with a big build up (lunchtime)
- full body seizure (5pm?)
- another full body seizure (5.30pm)
- seizure, eyes rolled back, fully stiff (5.45pm)
- seizure, bad (6pm?)

**Thursday 22/04/21**

- short seizure (7.35am)
- absences throughout day
- absence with teacher (3pm)
- small seizure (4/5pm)
- long seizure 6pm (unsure of what type)
- seizure, fell to floor (8pm, short but very shaky)

**Friday 23/04/21**

- hands paralysed/rigid (thumbs unlocked)
- absences all day
- 10 minute faint (2pm, friend timed on watch)
- under 5 mins faint (2.30pm)
- long absence (4-5 mins, with teacher, big build up)
- x2 faint on office sofa (2.45-3pm)
- seizure (4/5pm, lowered to floor)
- seizure (8.40pm)

**Saturday 24/04/21**

- seizure (afternoon maybe 4/5pm?)
- passed out a few times throughout the day
- absences periodically

**Sunday 25/04/21**

- absence/partial seizure (1.15pm)

- seizure - started from jaw (1.30pm)
- absence seizures throughout afternoon
- seizure - about 2 mins? (8.30pm)
- seizure - fell to floor (8.50pm?)
- seizure - fell again trying to get back up (8.55pm?)
- seizure - got onto bed just before (10pm)


And there's one week of life with FND!

I'm exhausted just thinking about it. I'm sure it may come as a shock to some of you reading this, but this is truly what my life looked like when my symptoms were unmanaged during exams. My diary entries became increasingly confusing to read because I often couldn't remember what had happened or the timing of episodes, therefore my days and weeks blurred together.

It became difficult for me to do anything independently in 2021 because my physical health was incredibly debilitating. A lot of the time, I couldn't stay conscious and had body parts which didn't work. My mum helped me get dressed in the mornings, I couldn't get up the stairs to our bathroom, and I never saw my friends outside of school due because of being too unwell or the activities being inaccessible.

I also couldn't cook at all due to my tics—it wasn't safe for me to hold a knife. I struggled to write neatly as my tics ripped up my pages in my schoolbooks and my hands ticced too much for me to write more than a word at a time. Since being young, I've prided myself on my perfectionist, colour-coded work and my small, even handwriting, so this was a very upsetting progression for me to accept.


My whole life consisted of symptoms, school work, sleeping and then posting some videos on social media to try to advocate for what was happening to me. It was a low and difficult year; I felt discouraged and hopeless on nearly all days during my last two years of secondary school. I'd lost all the normal aspects of a teen's social life due to Covid and my health struggles, and every day felt like an enormous battle just to make it through.

If you're suffering from a chronic illness, disability, or health condition (maybe you have FND too), then please know that it *can* get better with time, adaptations and avoiding triggers. Those hopeless, long days won't last forever, even though it feels like there's no way out in the moment.

I wouldn't have believed you if you told me what my life looks like whilst writing this book, because it looks vastly different from my teen years. I'm currently self-employed as a content creator, disability advocate and writer whilst working on this book. I don't attend school or college anymore (and decided not to go to university) which means that my symptoms aren't triggered every single day—this has made the biggest difference out of anything else.

~

Although my time in secondary school was really hard, I did find some things which helped to make it through exams, so I'd like to share my tips for navigating school with Tourette's or a chronic illness. I want to share with you all the accommodations I had during my GCSE exams, because I did (thankfully) achieve the grades I'd hoped for.

Firstly, I did my GCSEs in 2021, meaning Covid and lockdown changed our entire experience. Due to having missed months of school during lockdowns, the exam boards significantly cut content down to make up for this.

We also didn't sit our exams in the hall as planned, and we swapped to teacher-assessed grades for our year group. This meant I didn't have to sit any full-length exams or spend months revising, like students normally do before GCSEs in England. This was an absolute miracle in my case, because I didn't perform as well in exams as I usually did in lessons.

As somebody with Tourette's, sitting exams can feel impossible. Our tics often worsen with the stress of impending nerves, the quiet environment is impossible to stay silent in, and the constant movements and noises of our tics make it difficult to concentrate.

It was almost impossible for me to sit an exam when I was in secondary school, because my tics were in such a severe phase that I couldn't hold a pen without throwing it across the room! My tics scrunched the pages in my books, ripped up the exam papers and scribbled through words just after I'd finished writing them. It was unbelievably frustrating as somebody who just wanted to work hard and show the teachers how clever I *could* be when my brain actually allowed me to do the work.

In the end, they determined our grades using lots of mini-assessments which were sat in classes, though I completed these in a room by myself so I didn't disturb anybody. Our papers were also split into sections, meaning we only did one part of an exam at a time.

I studied as hard as I could to learn all the information at home, away from the noisy, stressful environment of the classroom. I'd be lying if I said this wasn't difficult to manage, but I do want to say that it *is* possible to study and get the grades you're capable of if accommodations are put in place to help you get there. I had to give up a *lot* of socialising in order to concentrate the little energy I had on my schoolwork, but this did make it possible to get my grades, so it was worth it in the end.

The main reason I made it through my GCSEs was due to my exam accommodations, which you can apply for if you have a disability or learning disability which prevents you from sitting an exam in the same way as everybody else.

For my exams, I applied for a **separate room** due to my tics being very disruptive. This took the pressure off me worrying about distracting other people. I also had the option to type my exams, which made writing a lot more accessible when my hands locked up from my FND, or when my motor tics wouldn't let me hold a pen.

Additionally, I had **25% extra time** on my exams, meaning I had a lot more time to let out my tics or work slowly when I wasn't feeling the best with my health. It took a lot longer to write sentences with tics scribbling out words, or my hand twitching upwards every time I tried to touch my pen to the paper.

Another *vital* adaptation we put in place was **rest breaks**. If you have any kind of seizure or fainting disorder like I do, then it may be helpful to have rest breaks so you can step outside and take a breather when your symptoms flare up. I find that my brain fog progressively worsens the longer I sit and concentrate for, so taking a walk around the block mid-way through an exam gave me time to stretch my legs, get some fresh air and also let any tics out that I'd been suppressing.

You can ask for other adaptations if needed, like somebody to **scribe** for you if you struggle to write or type. My exams weren't "official" GCSE exams, therefore I had permission to **play instrumental music** in my separate room, giving me relaxing input in the background. Music massively helps my tics, so this was a big relief for me! It nearly halves the amount of tics I have when I simply play music in the background of tasks, so whether it's studying or classwork, I always have my headphones plugged in.

These adaptations can be put in place using an **EHCP** (Education Health and Care Plan) or a care plan formed with your school and teachers, and there are equivalents of this in most countries.

"An Education, Health and Care plan (EHCP) is a legal document which describes a child (or young person's aged up to 25) special educational needs, the support they need, and the outcomes they would like to achieve."
   - Council for Disabled Children

An EHCP is intended for those who need more support than is available through the school's special educational needs department. A legal EHCP can be difficult to apply for, however they can provide speech and language therapy, occupational therapy, physiotherapy, one-to-one support from a teaching assistant, and other therapies and accommodations that are specific to your disability.

In my case, the learning support department at my school helped set up an internal care plan with my teachers, which we forwarded to every member of staff so they knew of my situation and needs. In a lot of cases, this is enough support for many of us if set up alongside applications for exam accommodations.

Schools can set up a care plan for any child or young person with a significant and long-term special educational need or disability. Tourette's and FND both qualify for this because these are neurological disabilities which significantly affect my life and my ability to learn. Other reasons someone may need a care plan or exam accommodations may include: dyslexia, ADHD, autism, cerebral palsy, down syndrome, epilepsy, severe anxiety and many other disorders or conditions.

You may be questioning, why this would actually help?

Having a plan (either with your school or as a legal document) means that all your needs are formally recognised and sent to your teachers—whether that's physical accessibility, learning disability needs or mental health adjustments. This is essential when applying for exam accommodations, and usually helps with getting day-to-day support and understanding too. This document can also help provide evidence of your needs when applying for benefits like Disability Living Allowance, PIP, Child Benefits, or Carers Allowance.

Speaking up and having your needs on paper can make an enormous difference when asked to provide evidence of your struggles, so I'd highly suggest sending an email or contacting your school to set this up!

~

Here is a summarised list of my top tips for surviving GCSEs or A-Levels with Tourette's, because I know there are many of you out there who are going through this tricky period. There are lots more accommodations than just the ones listed here, and support looks different for different conditions, so make sure to test and find what works for *you*. Everybody works differently!

## MY GUIDE TO EXAMS WITH TOURETTE'S:

1. **Try not to worry.** This seems counter-intuitive because, of *course* we all worry about our grades when we feel the pressure of a formal exam—but trust me when I say that these grades don't define your entire life. It won't be a disaster if you don't get the grade you hoped for; there are always other options. You are not a failure if you don't get the top academic grades, because there are so many other qualities to a person

than just academic ability, and these are often more important.

2. **Set up a care plan with your school.** If you don't have one already, making a care plan (or applying for an EHCP) can be useful when explaining to both your school and the exam board about your disability. You can add any struggles you have or symptoms which may inhibit your ability to focus or complete work, and this can be sent to all your teachers to ensure they're educated on your needs.

3. **Try to seek a diagnosis.** If you're struggling with an undiagnosed disability, then please know that you are completely valid! Your struggles are real, you deserve just as much support as somebody who is diagnosed, and you will get answers with time. But I'm afraid to say, having no diagnosis does make it more difficult to formally apply for adaptations in legal exams. Exam boards often request medical notes or doctor's letters to prove you have a diagnosis, so it's a good idea to speak to your GP and get this process started as early as possible to ensure you have the help you need when exams do roll around.

4. **Apply for exam adaptations.** Whether it's extra time, a separate room, a computer, or a scribe, having the right adaptations can make the difference between passing exams and failing them. You deserve an equal chance at performing to the best of your ability, and your disability shouldn't set you at a disadvantage. Even if it seems scary, please try to advocate for yourself and voice your needs! You never know how much it could help you.

5. **Use music when studying.** I've always found that music helps me to concentrate, and as I said before, it's one of the most effective ways to manage tics. Try playing some background music that can relax you

without being distracting, and see whether it helps you to complete work without tics getting in the way. If you're doing in-class exams (where the teacher is in control rather than the exam board), then you could ask to can play instrumental music during the test. It's better to ask and be rejected than to suffer in silence and never know whether it could have helped.

6. **Fidget toys** are a life-saver. Whether you struggle with writing tics or not, you've probably heard of fidget toys and how much they can help keep your brain busy in a way that simultaneously allows you to concentrate more. It sounds silly, but having a distraction in one hand actually allows me to concentrate *more* on what I'm doing! Having fidget toys, a ring to play with, spinners, or a squishy on my desk whilst working helps to reduce the amount of physical tics I have in my hands. This makes it easier to write without scribbling on the page and in addition to helping my tics, it calms my noisy, whirring head too.

7. **Track your triggers.** Whether it's sugar, caffeine, stress, friendships, or your morning routine before an exam, keeping track of tic triggers is essential if you want to spot patterns and reduce possible tic attacks. I found that socialising before an exam made my tics a lot more active, because other people or conversations usually trigger them. To combat this, I listened to calm music and sat on my own before exams rather than with friends—this helped me feel much more relaxed and prepared me for concentrating on my work.

8. **Practice!** I know you don't want to hear this, but practising exams and sitting in that same environment over and over again is the only way you're going to get used to it. The more comfortable and natural you feel in exam conditions, the less your tics will act up

due to stress. I completed all my in-class assessments in the same room that my official GCSEs would be in, therefore I was already used to the setup way before sitting my actual exams. I knew the whole setup, where I'd be sitting, where the clock was, how far away fresh air would be for when I need a break, and so on. This helped in *many* more ways than one— because I'm autistic, I need a lot of familiarity and routine, so practising in the same room made me feel much more confident.

Puberty is a common period where tics heighten for people with Tourette's, meaning it's common to be at your most active during this exam period. Many people with TS can relate and say that during school, their tics were at their most frequent and most severe. This was definitely true for me, and I think just being in school environments (with people who intentionally triggered my tics) made them a lot more active too.

School is a tricky and often very triggering environment to be in, so be patient with yourself and allow for a lot of rest in between exams or school days. You can only do how much you can do, so don't push yourself beyond your limits just to "keep up" with what other people around you are doing. It's better to go at your own pace and get all the accommodations you need, rather than spending years rushing around and ending up in burnout like many of us late-diagnosed neurodivergent people have done.

# FOURTEEN
# MY HEALTH'S DECLINE

With the added pressure of exams, my health took a turn for the worst towards the end of year eleven (age 15-16). It became extremely difficult to stay in school: my body paralysed or locked up on more days than not, and I had multiple seizures every single day.

Sometimes, after seizure episodes, my teachers had to help me along the corridors and into my mum's car. As time passed and my symptoms became more debilitating, my legs became more and more affected after episodes, meaning it was increasingly difficult to get around.

After a few seizures one day, I was in my deputy-headteacher's office lying down on her sofa. After a while, she came in with one of the learning support staff and they both helped me up and told me that my mum was outside, ready to take me home. I felt so drowsy that I didn't know exactly what was going on. My head felt like it was constantly spinning and my days blurred together when symptoms were frequent.

I remember standing in the corridor, my feet turning inwards and dragging along the floor as I tried to take steps forward—

my legs just wouldn't do what I told them. It was like trying to stand on your feet when you've been sitting for too long and get pins and needles. You know that awful feeling when you get a completely dead leg and can't figure out if your toes are touching the floor or not, because you can't feel it? That's sort of what it feels like.

I reached out my hand and used the wall to steady myself, but I kept dropping and eventually fell all the way to my knees on the floor. I must have had a few absence seizures because I don't remember the time in between the office and corridor—I only remember my teachers picking me up underneath my arms and carrying me along the corridor, one on each side of me.

Looking back on this shortly after, I felt so embarrassed. I couldn't fathom the thought of people seeing teachers carry me out of school, my feet dragging on the floor and my face distant as I fell in and out of consciousness.

It felt so vulnerable knowing I'd been in that state and couldn't do anything about it. My teachers had witnessed it, and all the people in the school had seen me fainted or limping down corridors at some point. I felt defeated, because I didn't want this life for myself, but I couldn't do anything to change it.

Denial is a huge process which most disabled people go through at some point in their journey. With changing symptoms and sometimes very sudden onsets, our debilitating health can be extremely jarring to cope with. It's so difficult to wrap your head around going from being a normal teenager who wants to fit in and party with their friends, to one who is physically carried out of school because their body won't let them stand up or stay conscious.

I still grieve my "healthy" body and a life without disability; it wouldn't be natural if at least a *part* of me didn't wish I could go back to having no health problems. But I have now accepted that this is a part of me, and what's done is done. This is the life I've been dealt and I'm going to make the most of every single moment I can!

My experiences can't be undone—you can't unmake a memory—but I've definitely found ways to re-arrange my thoughts and perspective over the years.

Yes, I wish I could run and travel and work a full-time job, and do all the other things my conditions make it difficult to do… but I'm also happy where I am.

I'm happy with my new-growing confidence in my disability. I'm happy with my extremely strong passion for advocacy, my love for researching and finding out about different conditions. I'm happy with the rainbow details I've decorated my wheel-chair with, because it lets me feel like myself despite the obvious symbol of being disabled. I'm happy with my friends and support system within the disabled community. I'm happy with my life, even with the challenges my health causes.

You *can* be disabled and happy.

You *can* be disabled and beautiful.

You *can* be disabled and talented.

And you *can* be disabled and live a rewarding life.

Although developing my conditions made my life quite horrendous for a while, it did teach me a lot of things about the world, about perspective, and about myself. I've learned that I'm pretty damn resilient! I can have a lot of challenges thrown at me, and I will still get through them. And I will always come out of the other side with a smile on my face—even if it disappeared during the messy process of coping.

I'm proud to be sharing my story. I don't feel too vulnerable, or unworthy because of my conditions or my disabilities any more. They don't define me, but they *are* a huge part of my life and identity, therefore they play a big role in how I live my life!

If you don't have a disability, I hope this chapter makes you think about what it can feel like to develop one. Try to consider what people in your life may be going through if they have a chronic illness or disability, and what you could do to help support them.

If you're reading this and you are disabled, then YOU ARE SMASHING IT!!! You are strong, and whatever your body is throwing at you right now, I hope there are ways to adapt so you can continue to live in a way that suits you. You will find love and happy moments in the chaos of disabled life. Living a full and happy life won't always feel unachievable or impossible—this just looks different for everybody.

~

After months of symptoms and my worsening physical state, my brain continued to throw challenges at me. It became harder and harder to go to school, until I eventually couldn't make it there at all.

In the past, I've always been the type of student to *never* miss a day unless my mum forced me to stay off sick—I didn't want to miss any lessons or fall behind—but suddenly I couldn't even get out of bed, never mind attend lessons. I couldn't get myself up the stairs to my bathroom, I couldn't shower, I couldn't move my my arms or legs over half of the time, and my physical capabilities became very limited.

My life shrunk to a small portion of what it had been before… and this was when we decided I needed a mobility aid to help me get outside and living again.

This is when the option of using mobility aids came up. I'd used crutches a couple times before, and with the development of my Tourette's and neurological symptoms, we'd collected a plethora of different braces, supports, splints, ice packs and every other aid under the sun. That was, except a wheelchair.

Deciding to get a wheelchair was a tricky decision mentally, because I still had all the internalised stigma surrounding wheelchairs at this point. Many questions came up, which some of you may have thought to yourself before.

*Would I have to use this forever?*
*Am I "stuck" in a wheelchair?*
*Am I giving up on myself?*
*What if people think I'm lazy? Or faking?*
*Will people think of me as the same person as before?*
*But… don't only paralysed people need wheelchairs?*

But, I also had to ask myself some even **more** important questions.

*What if I can go to school again?*
*Will this help my energy levels from now on?*
*What if this gives me my life back?*
*What if I can still enjoy living, even with all of my symptoms?*

Somewhere in between speaking to my Tourette's friends in group chats, researching online, and speaking with my mum... we finally ordered a wheelchair.

My first feeling was relief when I finally sat in the chair and managed to roll around my bedroom. I remember using my fluffy rug to decorate the seat, and using one of my bed cushions to make the seat more comfortable since this was only a basic folding wheelchair.

The next day, I used my crutches to get out of the house (since we have steps to get into both the porch *and* the front door) and my mum loaded my new wheelchair into the car before driving me to school. We had to arrange a meeting with my subject teachers and the deputy head-teacher to create a safety plan. There was a lot more to consider than I'd initially thought, and I immediately felt overwhelmed. This is where my first experience of accessibility issues began.


My school had stairs... a *lot* of stairs. We had no lifts, and there wasn't always a route which didn't involve steps, so this meant I couldn't properly get around the school, even with my new wheelchair. We had to plan for a teacher or a friend to always stay with me for safety, in addition to always bringing my crutches so I could get up the stairs.

Every time my lesson was upstairs, I had to drag myself up onto my crutches—despite having wobbly or locked legs—and make my way up the steps either on my bum or with somebody helping me up. Another friend had to carry my wheelchair up the stairs and set it at the top, so I could get back in when I'd climbed the steps.

It was a very tedious process, and I had to leave all my lessons early to make sure I had enough time to commute without people knocking me over or staring. I also struggled to propel myself in this wheelchair because the armrests were very high, so it was nearly impossible to reach over and wheel myself for any length of time. Despite this being frustrating, it did result in some fun memories of friends pushing my chair around!

A positive memory of this time involved a friend who supported me when my health became an enormous battle. She was very understanding and accepting of my health problems and helped me get around in my wheelchair as much as possible.

We'd leave lessons early, and I'd always choose her to escort me if we were in the same lesson. We'd zoom down the corridors with her pushing me as fast as possible without tipping me out. These moments were little snippets of laughter in a difficult time, so I'm really grateful I had people around me to help me through.

However, not everybody knew how to act around my new wheels and I faced a lot of stares and questions, especially in the first few months. Nobody else in my school used a wheelchair—I was the first, meaning everybody wanted to look and see what it was. People in the corridors stared a lot and since they already knew me from my Tourette's videos online, they started to think I was pretty weird.

On my first school day using my wheelchair, I remember wheeling into a maths lesson after everybody had sat down and the path was clear. My teacher moved my seat to the back of the room (near the door) for easier access, and made sure I was sitting next to a friend so I felt more comfortable. Being at the back of the classroom was comforting because everyone's chairs faced forwards, therefore they wouldn't be able to stare. However, as soon as we all got into the room, everybody started whispering or asking me questions.

I remember hearing one person say to his friend, "What happened to her?!" before another friend gave them a warning look and quickly shushed them. It felt like I was an unspeakable topic—people thought it was so terrible that I had to use a wheelchair. They asked me why I needed it, and people pulled sad faces or said they were really sorry that I was "stuck" in a wheelchair. This struck me as odd, because the chair had given me some independence *back*. Wasn't it a good thing?

This was the first time I experienced the negative attitude people have towards wheelchair users and people who use mobility aids. I quickly learned that some people don't value or respect you *nearly* as highly as non-disabled people, and sometimes stop treating you like a capable person.

People didn't include me in as many conversations (even though my social skills hadn't changed) and people seemed to look away when I met their gaze. It was like people didn't know how to talk to me at all anymore!

I tried to let people in by telling them some of my story or my symptoms, but this often ended in more sympathy I wasn't looking for. I wanted people to understand and then move on and treat me as normal—I didn't want to wallow or treat my symptoms like something that *had* to define me.


One day during morning registration, I let some classmates try out my wheelchair after they'd asked a few times. I felt a little nervous because I didn't like people touching my stuff (another autistic tendency I still struggle with to this day), but I said yes because they were the "popular" kids and I wanted to be friendly to them.

They played around and some of them saw the "fun" in using a wheelchair, asking if I could do a wheelie and similar questions which, surprisingly, I didn't mind. It was a pleasant change from the negative talk I usually got, so I welcomed it!

However, one of those classmates frowned almost immediately after sitting in my chair and after wheeling forwards and backwards, they commented on how difficult it was to push. They said out loud that they felt uncomfortable and felt "so disabled" sitting in that chair, and they didn't know how people could ever do that. I wasn't sure how to respond, so I told them that I didn't have a choice—this was just the card I'd been dealt in life—and smiled before trying to move on.

People often have very different responses to my mobility aids, but at the time of writing this, I've become really confident in my wheelchair—which is now a custom-fit chair with rainbow wheels and a cool checker-board calf strap across the front. I love making myself feel colourful and treating my wheelchair as an extension of me, rather than something clinical or negative.

I love my wheelchair! It gives me access to the outside world when my body isn't strong enough to hold me up for very long. It allows me to go further distances, and it gets me out of the house during flare-ups.

If somebody needs to use a mobility aid (whether it's a walking stick, crutches, a wheelchair or something else) please help them feel comfortable. Make them feel respected, and don't treat them any differently just because they need an aid to give them more freedom.

People who use mobility aids don't need your sympathy, but we do need understanding and accessibility. We need step-free access to public places. We need seating available so we can sit down when we don't feel well. We need carers access if we can't go to places on our own and need to be escorted. We need access to the same opportunities everybody else would have in their daily lives, and to do that, society needs to make our world more accessible for *everyone*.

Using a wheelchair felt like an enormous leap for me, and it was absolutely terrifying as a teenager in public secondary school. I felt incredibly anxious that people would judge me, and some of them did. The world isn't always accepting, accessible or under-standing, even though it definitely should be.

Acceptance wasn't a smooth journey and it was a hard, long process to adjust to my new normal. Being a wheelchair user changed how I view my life and a lot of society—but getting my wheelchair was a step that I 100% needed to take.

$$\sim$$

Despite all of my struggles adapting to my health conditions, I did gain some positives from the situation too! One secondary school achievement that I'm proud of, is delivering a speech to my entire class about Tourette's syndrome.

For my GCSE spoken language assessment, we had to prepare a presentation on a topic of our choice. Immediately, I knew I wanted to talk about my neurological condition and I felt incredibly excited to have an opportunity to educate people. I spent hours researching (though I already knew a lot of the facts by this point!) and I prepared a power-point and flash cards. I rehearsed my speech again and again, recording myself to see how long it would take and ensuring I could stand up and talk for that long without triggering my health issues.

I'm not going to lie, I was absolutely terrified! My hands were shaking, and my tics were active before I started my speech because my nerves shot through the roof. I handed out Tourette's Action (our UK charity for Tourette's syndrome) information cards to my peers and then stood up at the front of the class-room, waiting to begin.

My tics took a few minutes to calm down before I got "in the zone" and concentrated as hard as I could. One of my best friends helped to set up my phone on her desk at the front of the classroom so I could record my speech and later share it on social media if it went well. I'd asked my teacher for permission beforehand, and I'm so glad I did because it's now been seen by hundreds of thousands of you!

If you're a teacher reading this and you'd like to educate your class on TS or ableism within schools, then feel free to watch my class presentation on my YouTube channel or maybe even share it with your pupils. I hope it can help more people understand what Tourette's syndrome is really like underneath the stigma and misconceptions.

I successfully completed my speech the whole way through, only ticcing a few times vocally because my tics lessen significantly when I'm engrossed in something I feel passionate about. I relaxed into the flow of my sentences and delivered probably the best speech of my life—I'm really proud of doing this despite feeling so anxious.

I hope this can inspire some of you who have anxiety, tics, or Tourette's and show you that you *can* do things you're afraid of. Tics aren't something to be ashamed of, and even though standing up in front of your class is pretty terrifying, you should be proud to be talking about things that mean a lot to you!

Doing the hard thing is sometimes the best thing we can do for our mental strength. Pushing ourselves out of our comfort zones can feel impossible in the moment, but I assure you that it helps to build strength in the long run. If you have a goal that you've been avoiding because you're scared or nervous, then I challenge you to face it (or make a plan to start building up to it) after reading this book. Even if it's something as "small" as stepping outside for a few minutes and then coming back in, I'm proud of you. I'm already sending virtual hugs to any of you who are going to face your fears today, or this week, or this year... you are amazing, and you can do this.

If you have Tourette's and would like to tell your class about your condition, prepare a speech, or share your story, then I do recommend it! If you can put together an informative presentation and ask your teacher to show it to your class, it could help somebody learn something new about neurological disabilities.

On the other hand, if you don't like sharing your story with others, then it's completely okay for you not to. Disclosing your medical history, conditions and your journey is *your* choice; you don't owe anybody an explanation. Ever.

Another positive memory from this time actually *includes* my tics! Despite my Tourette's causing a lot of stress and inconvenience, a lot of my vocal tics at school were quite funny. They sometimes said whole sentences and often finished other people's sentences, which definitely gave my friends a good laugh on many occasions.

A frequently amusing lesson was my maths class, because most of my friends at the time were also in my class. Back then, one of my most common tics was saying "the chickens" in a high-pitched voice, and this always made people laugh. I also said "it's the chickens, Mrs Tweedy" which you might recognise from the film *Chicken Run*! This is an example of an echolalia tic, where I hear something on a TV show or from somebody else saying it, then my tics repeat it involuntarily.

Sometimes certain tics become common phrases, and I say them every single day, more than any other tic—this has happened with many different tics throughout my years of having TS. Tics usually come and go in phases of different words or movements being the most frequent ones, but sometimes I may only tic something once.

I began ticcing words and phrases about chickens more and *more* and *more* until my brain had almost come up with a storyline for these chickens! I had different phrases that connected to other tic phrases, forming complete sentences.

People in that class began to notice this and whenever I started to tic something, we'd all wait to see whether my tics would reveal something new about these "chickens" (me included, because I didn't know what I was about to say). It was pretty hilarious! Even my teacher laughed at my tics—he did try to hold it in, but none of us could help it!

The things my tics said made that class feel very light-hearted and fun, so I don't mind those tics at all. It's the painful physical tics or the highly offensive verbal phrases that I really don't like.

Funny vocal tics are just one small, light-hearted part of my condition, and not everybody with Tourette's had words and phrases as tics. Vocal tics can also be squeaks, grunts, animal noises and other sounds.

Please remember that although individual tics can be funny, Tourette's is not a funny condition. It may be okay to laugh along with a person's tics if they say that you can, but be mindful that there's a lot we have to deal with behind the scenes —tics can cause a lot of discomfort and inconvenience.

Some of my classmates started to intentionally trigger my tics once they became more familiar with the words I frequently said. If they found a phrase funny, they'd say it over and over again until I involuntarily repeated it (thanks, echolalia). This became very boring and frustrating within only a few weeks of being back in school, and as the months went by, I really despised having echolalia tics in classes.

I felt completely out of control, because all I wanted to do was fight back and prove people wrong, but I physically *couldn't* stop my tics from repeating what people said. I couldn't choose whether or not to tic those things, so more often than not, the people "won" and my tics provided the source of laughter people were seeking.

I quickly felt a bit like a class clown, without ever signing up for the role. I didn't want to be constantly laughed at. I didn't like shouting funny things in silent classrooms, even if it entertained other people. On the outside, I was confident and involuntarily outspoken, but on the inside, my anxiety was getting progressively worse.

When you're around anybody with tics or Tourette's, please take this into account and consider their feelings. Do they want to be the centre of jokes all the time? Would they prefer it if you ignored their tics rather than played into them? Can you do anything to make them feel less exposed or vulnerable?

If you're a teacher, ask yourself what you can put in place to make the classroom a little safer for your students with tics or other outwardly shown disabilities. Can you educate the class to help them to understand why laughing at people can be hurtful? Could you talk to your disabled students and make systems they feel comfortable with? Can you create a safe space for that student to use, or give them a pass to leave the classroom when needed?

There are *always* ways to change our environments and put accommodations in place to make disabled people feel more safe. There are *always* ways you can change how you act around others if it's making them feel uncomfortable.

Ask your disabled classmates or co-workers how they feel about your interactions, and whether you can change anything to make them feel more accepted. Make a conscious effort *not* to make jokes about disabilities. Stand up for something people are making fun of. Try to educate people on a topic they misunderstand.

There are unlimited ways we can be better allies to the disabled community, and even minor changes can lead to making a bigger difference. Being a bystander is definitely easier than being an advocate, but if everybody changed *one* small thing at a time, the world could become a more accepting and safe place for people who are different.

# FIFTEEN
# THE HIGHS & LOWS OF GOING VIRAL

Alongside my health, I faced big challenges in other ways too. My life was changing rapidly and part of this was my online life. My videos were reaching people all over the world, which produced a chance to educate even more people on my conditions. I'm forever grateful for this opportunity and where it's led me, but one difficulty this brought me… was hate comments.

I hadn't had many awful or negative comments since my bullying experiences earlier in secondary school, so these hate comments came as a bit of a shock. I'd received a few "faker" comments in my months of posting online, but nothing prepared me for the increase in DMs and comments I received after my Covid Test video.

After going viral—and hitting over 90 million views—that video brought millions of people to my page who had no idea what Tourette's or FND was, or even what a disability was! Many people came from drastically different cultural or spiritual backgrounds, meaning every follow had a unique opinion on what Tourette's was and how to approach it. As you can probably guess, this resulted in some bizarre comments.

I've been told many times that I "need an exorcism" or that I'm "possessed by dark spirits" even though these ideas are about two *centuries* old and scientifically proven to be inaccurate. Here's an exact quote of a comment I received:

> You are giving yourself over to demonic oppression and have opened the doors to possession. I recommend you look up some testimonies of occult practitioners and mediums who found God.

Tourette's was discovered in the late 19th century, after a French neurologist named Gilles de la Tourette published a paper in 1885 on a rare condition which caused involuntary movements and swearing. Before this discovery and the medical knowledge and scientific technologies of today, people with Tourette's were thought to be mentally ill, lacking in self-control, or quite simply possessed.

Until the early 1970s, psychoanalysis was the most common intervention for Tourette's, but we now know that tics are caused by misfired signals in the brain. They stem from a part of the brain called the basal ganglia, which helps to control bodily movements. They can't be *cured* by any known treatment at the time of writing this.

There are medications which can help some people with Tourette's, and there are ways of managing triggers and reducing stress to help reduce tic activity, but tics aren't something that needs to be cured purely because they're different.

Tics can cause pain and uncomfortable situations, but I believe the biggest struggle is the way people react to us! We need to view Tourette's as something to accept and learn to live *with*, rather than a problem to be solved, hated or avoided at all costs. This only makes people with tics feel like they're undeserving of support or respect in "normal" society.

People with Tourette's are NOT possessed, and we can't be cured by simply reading a religious piece of text or by praying to be healed. Trust me, if we could, I'd have done it! Tourette's doesn't have a cure, but it's something that most of us learn to adapt and live with. We need acceptance, understanding and to be accommodated for in the world; we don't need to be exorcised, prayed for or hidden away.

During my rapid increase of viewers, another tricky situation was caused by people's reactions to offensive tics or racial slurs. This topic is so incredibly difficult to navigate (and to even talk about) but that's exactly why I want to include it in my book.

Contrary to popular misconceptions, people with Tourette's *don't* tic what we think. We can't control it, and most of the time our brain says the exact *opposite* thing to what we should say in situations, meaning it's often the most socially unacceptable thing to say in that scenario. This doesn't originate from a specific thought in our heads, and tics aren't usually a conscious thought at all! Of course, visual stimuli or the topic of conversation can influence which tics we have, but this isn't intentional on our part.

When trying to practice racial sensitivity and avoid using slurs, coprolalia tics can become a huge issue for people with Tourette's—it can even be dangerous. I have experienced inappropriate or offensive tics in the past, and I quickly learned with my growing audience that people don't understand this at all.

No matter how hard I tried to educate people on coprolalia or why my brain says these things, I received hundreds of comments calling me racist, homophobic (despite being openly queer myself!) and many things I won't repeat.

This left me feeling disheartened and though I never shared this online, I almost quit. I nearly gave up this entire part of my life—the advocacy I have such a strong passion for—because I couldn't get through to people. I didn't know how to help people understand and how to move forward with sharing my condition. I didn't know how to navigate having a socially unaccepted disability that I couldn't control.

It's important for people to know that Tourette's isn't controllable. Our tics can happen anywhere, with anybody, and at any time. This means we don't have the privilege of deciding who can hear our tics or the privilege to refrain from saying offensive things around people who may feel personally targeted by them.

I would *never* condone voluntarily saying a slur or offensive phrase against another person or minority, so *please* don't do this if you can help it and you don't have Tourette's. There is so much hate in this world and we should be kind to others as often as we can; we never know what people might be going through.

But this is where the dilemma comes into play... We need to practice sensitivity around other cultures, religions, races and minorities, but this isn't always a choice for people with Tourette's when we have involuntary tics. We don't have the option to avoid saying words that may hurt others, even when we don't want to say anything at all.

People with Tourette's are not horrible or insensitive people, and people should give us space to let our tics out, because this prevents painful build-ups and tic attacks. As a society, we need to understand that tics are involuntary so that people feel safe enough to let their tics out in public. We shouldn't have to hide or be afraid that people will misunderstand us or categorise us as something we're not, purely due to our condition.

On the flip side, there is a small risk that *some* people may take advantage of this acceptance and use Tourette's as an excuse to use vulgar language, therefore I do understand why people are wary or quick to judge.

Tourette's is often misunderstood as an "excuse" to swear or say what's on our minds, which is completely inaccurate! This is a misconception that causes damage to people in the Tourette's community every single day. We work incredibly hard to educate people and make sure the world knows that TS isn't a "swearing pass" or a free ticket to say what we think without consequences, so this misconception threatens to undo the work of so many advocates and charities.

Please never allow jokes or misbeliefs about Tourette's to go uneducated, because they can be so harmful and often perpetuate the idea that our tics are what we are thinking.

There is no "right" or "wrong" way to deal with coprolalia, but my guidance is to be respectful whether you have tics yourself or you're witnessing somebody with tics. Offer kindness before you jump to conclusions or defensiveness, because more often than not, the person with tics is feeling more anxious and uncomfortable than bystanders are.

We don't want to hurt or offend anybody, so please research and really get to know people before leaving a comment online or assuming they truly think the negative things their tics say.

～

Despite learning to build walls between myself and the online world, some comments have really affected me in the past. I'm not easily upset by comments, and I can usually laugh at them rather than feel hurt, but this isn't the case for a lot of people online.

Keyboard warriors or cyberbullies are a very real threat, and some people can be truly awful when they think there are no consequences when commenting behind the safety of a screen. They leave hate comments on videos they've only seen a few seconds of, and frequently attack people for the way they look based on only one video. Comments like this usually come from uneducated, sad people who truly don't have anything nice to say; if you receive any negative comments, please report them and show them to somebody you can trust before deleting them. You deserve better!

I sometimes make the mistake of scrolling through the endless streams of comments on my videos—it's a deep hole to get caught up in. I want to share some comments I've received in the past few weeks to show how the internet can treat people and to prove that comments, more often than not, don't originate from any truth. I'll also comment after each one, dispelling the stigma and correcting factually-inaccurate parts of each comment to educate you and let you know that this is wrong.

If you ever receive a nasty comment either in person or online, please know that this is not your fault or anything you've done wrong.

> Why are you living such a miserable life. It's
> better to just die.

Nobody should ever be told they shouldn't be alive because they struggle with a disability. It makes me sad that some people in this world truly don't have enough hope that they believe being different is a life sentence. Disabled people deserve life. They deserve happiness, respect, and to *enjoy* their existence.

Suicide is a very prevalent and deadly threat. The latest UK suicide figures show that on average, just under 6,000 people take their own lives every year, which is around 15 people every single day. Large amounts of teens suffer from bullying either online or in schools, and this increases the likelihood of suicide. Disabled or neurodivergent people are also more likely to be targeted for being different, which can lead to people developing depression or even attempting to end their own lives.

This shouldn't be happening, but it goes unnoticed so often. People shouldn't be exposed to such hate simply by going online, but unfortunately we are. I try to make my corner of the internet a safe space as much as possible, but please take care and protect yourself by using privacy settings and limiting comments where you can.

> You're going to grow up and realize some day that you sucked all the emotional capacity out of your friends and family, and nobody will want to be around you.

This comment really struck home, because my anxiety likes to tell me I'm unwanted, and being autistic makes me feel like I don't (and will never) fit in anywhere I go. I now know that I'm loved and I *am* worthy of relationships, but I can definitely relate to all the disabled people who feel like they're a burden.

We already have unbearable symptoms to deal with which we can't control or get rid of—and this does produce a lot of stress for both us and the people around us. We need extra help, accommodations, and sometimes a lot of support from loved ones, which can make us feel like we're "hard work" or that we're a burden on our families or friends. But, trust me when I say that we are not.

You are not a burden. You deserve love and support, and having a disability doesn't make you a problem—no matter how big or small your support needs are.

> I have seen many cases of Tourette's and not once was it biting oneself and hitting a wall for hours. If she is that unable to control her body and is violent towards herself or others, then she shouldn't be in the general population.

This comment perfectly displays the massive stigma surrounding Tourette's that we touched on earlier: the belief that our tics are dangerous and reflect our thoughts or feelings. But again, this is not true! We cannot control our tics, but that doesn't make us dangerous to the population. It means we need extra support when our bodies are misfiring signals.

Isolating disabled people is ableism, and it is extremely harmful to our mental well-being. As a society, we should be implementing necessary adaptations to make disabled people feel comfortable, not pushing disabled people further away or into confinement.

Another misconception here is that every person with Tourette's looks the same, when in reality we all look completely different. If you've met one person with Tourette's, then you've met one person with Tourette's! This saying applies in many other circumstances, but it holds truthful here too. Knowing and seeing one person's presentation of symptoms doesn't make you an expert on the condition, because every person is different. Everybody's tics are unique, and many people have vastly different severities, ranging from being hardly noticeable to outsiders, to being severely debilitating or being deemed "socially unacceptable" to the general public.

"What if they just tied you up?"

Physically restraining somebody against their will is abusive behaviour, just as it would be in any other circumstance. Tics often worsen if the person is physically restricted or held down via any method, therefore tying somebody up in an attempt to stop their tics can actually cause a lot of harm and make the person's tics even more violent or persistent.

Tics *can* feel frustrating for people with Tourette's, and also for anybody who is repeatedly witnessing repetitive movements and sounds, but this does not give anybody an reason to physically restrain somebody and cause pain, purely to make other people feel more comfortable.

"Stop making fun of people with serious struggles. GET A LIFE or lose yours."

Now, this brings us back to the topic of bullying, because telling somebody to lose their life is never okay.

This is just one of *many* messages I've received telling me I either don't deserve to live, or that they believe I should end my life. It's saddening to think of people genuinely believing somebody shouldn't be alive, and it angers me to see this commented on real human being's social media pages. I am a human being. I am real, and I have feelings. I have a life—which I love—and I deserve to live it.

It will *never* be okay to tell somebody to lose their life, especially if that person is posting vulnerable content about their disability and trying to educate people!

If you ever receive a death threat, a message suggesting or idealising suicide, or telling you that you are unworthy, please know that this is not true and you do not deserve this. You are valuable and deserving of life, no matter what you've been through or any differences you may have.

Good people exist in this world if we search in between these nasty pockets of the internet, so please don't let comments and people like this determine how you treat or value yourself. It took me a long time to realise this and to respect myself, but I have truly learned that these comments don't reflect who I am as a person. They aren't truthful, they don't determine anything about me, they don't define my worth, and I don't have to accept them. And neither do you.

The pressures of maintaining an audience and posting the "correct" videos to please every single person (this is impossible, by the way) is a really heavy and stressful weight to carry at the age of fourteen or fifteen. It's a heavy weight to carry at any age!

I remember my mum being increasingly worried about my online presence and my videos going viral at a young age, but we talked through everything and she supported me—along with the rest of my family and friends—to help manage the new people, comments and feelings that were brought up. Having a support system and a team of people you can share information and thoughts with is essential when protecting your own mental health.

∼

One thing I don't think I'll ever quite get used to is being recognised in public! It seems absolutely unbelievable that people see me in the street or while I'm out shopping or attending an event, and come to ask for a photo with me. It truly makes my day when somebody smiles and tells me they like my content, because it's a reminder that my videos are having a positive impact on real people.

One day after finishing secondary school, I was walking through my town when two people recognised me. My face turned bright red as I smiled and thanked them for complimenting my content. I was incredibly awkward the first few times people came up to me because I have anxiety and I'm autistic, so I don't *actually* know how to talk to new people. However, over time I have gotten better at this and I'm hopefully much more exciting to chat to nowadays!

After making it across the town centre, I walked into McDonald's. As I stood in the queue, the worker recognised me from TikTok—I was so embarrassed! She told me that she liked my videos and that her daughter watched them too. I then walked up to the counter to get my food, and yet another follower came up and said hello!

This experience felt like a prank at first, because I couldn't fathom having so many people recognise me in one place. It's lovely to meet the real faces behind the numbers on the screen, but it can definitely be daunting too. It's intimidating knowing that people could recognise or take photos of you… even when you don't notice them.

The worst in-person interaction I had was at a bus station about two years ago. I was crossing the bus lanes to meet my friend on the other side when I heard laughing and shouting behind me. I turned around to see a group of younger teens pointing at me and saying things I couldn't quite hear.

I brushed this off with the assumption they were just having fun, but then they shouted my name. I didn't know them, so I was confused and tried to walk away. They started to follow me, shouting my name louder until I turned around and looked at them.

I suddenly realised they were filming me as they came closer, and this is where I panicked. Being in public already makes me nervous, so I struggled to catch my breath and felt the familiar signs of a panic attack approaching. They filmed me as I walked across the bus station until I reached my friend and explained what was happening.

It's scary being followed. I worried for days whether they'd post a video of me and I'd be tagged in it, though of course I'd done nothing wrong—I was only walking through the town centre!

If you ever see somebody you recognise from social media, please never film them without their consent! Most times, I'm happy to chat with people or take a photo if they ask, but to somebody with anxiety, situations like this can be frightening.

I hope this provides some insight into what it can be like from a creator's perspective in scenarios like this. When you're staring at or taking photos of somebody, think about their feelings and reconsider how you can make them feel more comfortable.

～

Phew! That was a fairly heavy segment—the internet can be a weird and pretty unsafe place if you venture outside of your community. But, alongside the negative pressure, anxiety, hate and a lot of judgemental people, there are also many benefits of going viral.

I've made lifelong friends, founded a community of people who all share their experiences and connect with each other, I've created a career for myself, found a passion in advocacy, photography, video editing, and if you're reading this, then I've successfully published my writing.

So many opportunities have emerged from the past few years, and it all started with me posting short, awkward videos on my personal TikTok account. If you've been here since the start, then I appreciate you so much—you're truly incredible.

And if you're new or reading this book without ever having seen my content, then hello and thank you!

I've definitely gained enough positive experiences to outweigh any problems or hate comments. My advocacy has been featured in the news, I've recorded podcasts, done countless interviews including platforms like BuzzFeed, and I even filmed a short documentary which was intimidating but such a cool experience!

I've also gained an entire community of like-minded people who love to talk about their differences, embracing disabled life while bringing others up and letting them know that they're not alone.

Many amazing friends have come from my time online, and I've since met some of them in person! Jess and Anouk are two friends I met through our shared experiences posting about our Tourette's. When I met my other friends Seren and Neve, I felt so accepted. We chatted and spent a whole day together, looking after one other whenever our tics got in the way, and they made sure I was safe during any seizures I had. Seren is also blind, so she showed us how to navigate using her cane, which brought a whole new element of education to our dynamic. I love meeting kind and interesting people who can relate to me in some ways, but also teach me so many new things too.

One group of amazing people who supported me through my online journey are my friends with Tourette's, starting with a group chat back in 2020. We spoke nearly every day at the beginning, and we still catch up with each other even now. I feel fully accepted and free to express myself when I'm talking to my friends in the Tourette's community, and since many of us make content to raise awareness, they're amazing at giving advice!

I have also met countless close friends through Tourette's Action events, so I highly recommend reaching out to charities or local support groups for any condition, difference or hobby you may have.

To any of the people I've mentioned in this chapter, I want you to know that I am so grateful to have you in my life, and meeting you guys felt like I finally had somebody who could understand me. Meeting people who have the same conditions as me—even if our journeys are very different—brings me a sense of belonging I'd never felt before.

I don't have to worry about my tics because I know my friends understand the pressures of socialising with Tourette's. I don't have to worry about how I look or how people will react to my seizures, because everybody in the community understands what I'm going through and knows exactly how to respond.

Communities for chronic illness, Tourette's, FND, autism and the general disabled or neurodivergent online space can be such a heart-warming and welcoming place if you find the right corner to settle in.

There are a great deal of resources, group chats, posts, videos, meet-ups and so many other ways to get involved and feel accepted. Tourette's Action holds retreats for people with Tourette's, and I've attended a few of these over the years. These have been incredible experiences which completely changed my entire perspective on my condition, but I will cover this more in later chapters.

No matter what condition or difference you may have, reach out to communities and support groups either online or locally. You never know what tips or support you could find!

# SIXTEEN
## STARTING COLLEGE

The whirlwind of my online life slowly calmed down over the summer before college. Whenever I felt well enough, I spent every day of that summer outside with my friends. I still struggled with my health a lot, but I still made the most of my time—and since I wasn't in school, it was much easier to manage my symptom triggers.

I remember having a fun, freeing couple of weeks despite having *many* friendship struggles and feeling like I didn't *quite* fit in. As usual, I couldn't keep up with the different groups or social occasions. I've always felt that I'm not on the "same level" as people the same age as me, and after researching about autism post-diagnosis, I discovered that this is common among autistic people!

I constantly feel too young compared to my peers: I don't like partying, going out late, drinking, I don't attend many social occasions, and I prefer to do my own hobbies and activities at home with a cup of tea. But similarly, I'm mentally "too old" or mature to fit in with my age group, meaning I'm constantly caught in the middle. Simultaneously too old and too young to fit in.

But recently, I've realised this is a common feeling that autistic people experience, and I've also learned that this is completely okay. You don't have to fit in or act the same way as people your age. If the stereotypical boxes don't fit you, then step out of the box and do your own thing!

It's okay to do what *you* like rather than what's expected of you as a teen or an adult—you don't have to feel guilty or weird for preferring different things! You don't have to change yourself to fit in with other groups of people, even if you desperately want them to like you. In my experience, trying to people please and doing your absolute best to fit in only results in failed friendships further down the line. You need to find those people who like who you are underneath, the ones who accept you without the mask—and trust me, they *are* out there.

It's taken me nineteen years to figure out how to be myself around people, and only recently have I actually found friendships where I feel comfortable and accommodated! It's a lengthy process and often results in losing people along the way, but the feeling of complete acceptance and joy when you do finally find your people is so worth it.

The summer before I started college, I tried incredibly hard to blend into a very sociable group, and although it worked for a while (I *did* have some fun days out), I eventually burned out, ending my streak of improved health *and* my friendships. My fainting episodes became more frequent and my friends were catching me right, left and centre during days at the park or while out shopping. My seizures were still quite active, though not as severe as during exams. But… this all changed when I started college, starting with our sign-up day.

When I applied for college and received my place, my year group had to visit the college buildings to register, do an interview, and take our ID photos. I thought this would go smoothly, but as you may have realised in the earlier pages of this book, nothing is ever simple when you throw health conditions in the mix.

The first hurdle appeared when I couldn't safely go into college alone because of seizure risks. My tics were also extremely active with the added nerves, so I needed support for this too. When I have very interruptive vocal tics, it becomes difficult to explain or advocate for myself, therefore I needed somebody to come and help advocate for me. My mum escorted me to college despite nobody else bringing a parent with them, which I knew made people look at me differently.

A strange feeling of inferiority washed over me that day, because this was supposed to be the start of my independent stage of life—the age where we learn to be adults and prepare for university—but I was still being escorted by a parent. However, my mum made me laugh a lot and I was relieved to have her there with me. She helped figure out where to go and re-directed questions or looks from people around us.

If you're neurodivergent in any way and need support, I'd highly recommend bringing somebody along if you can, because this can make you feel a lot less alone and vulnerable.

I first had to take an ID photo in the assembly hall—this took *many* takes before my tics stopped twitching my face or sticking my tongue out (the photographer's out-takes must have been quite hilarious). After completing some forms in the computer room, we entered a bigger room which was filled with people. I cringed as I recognised a few people from my previous school, and I also felt intimidated by the tables of teachers sat around the room peering at us.

I walked towards a kind-looking staff member—hoping she'd be understanding—and picked up a form to sign, sitting down in the middle of the room with everybody else. Although the other students only took a second to write their name, it took me over fifteen minutes! My tics were *really* active; I couldn't write because my tics wouldn't even let me get the pen to paper without my hand ticcing and jerking away. My mum actually had to write my signature for me in the end!

We organised for the learning support staff to conduct my spoken interview, so this went surprisingly well! The conversation naturally flowed, and I got on especially well with one of the female staff members who was really bright and bubbly. She made me laugh immediately, and she never failed to do so for the rest of my college experience. The learning support staff made my college feel like a safer place, even on the hardest days when I just wanted to go home and hide.

The first weeks of college were increasingly difficult. After only a few days, I knew surviving college was going to be really, *really* hard. Much like the transition between primary and secondary school, starting college was particularly tough for me due to all the sudden changes. As the unfamiliar environment sent me into a spiral, my anxiety peaked, my mental health plummeted, and the stress made me unable to function.

I now recognise this as an autistic struggle: being very sensitive to change. I struggle with even the smallest changes to my daily routine, therefore enormous life adjustments can trigger meltdowns and often cause a lot of stress and executive dysfunction.

In my first weeks of college, I suffered another friendship breakup which left me with nobody to eat lunch with or help me navigate when I got overwhelmed. I'd started in a new place, with new teachers, new subjects, new timetables, different lunches, no established safe spaces... and then I lost all of my friends too.

Everything went downhill as the stress of social struggles tipped my body over the edge, sending me into a full neurological flare-up. My body stopped working, my limbs wouldn't move properly, my hands and feet locked up in rigid positions, and I was hardly conscious due to constant episodes and seizures. My body basically stopped functioning altogether!

I didn't have friends to take me to lessons or lunch, so I began to close off from people. I spent my free time and social breaks in the learning support rooms, and I went home straight after my lessons finished. I stopped getting lunch at school because I couldn't manage the journey in my wheelchair and didn't want to face the rush of people on my own.

I didn't want to sit by myself, I couldn't open doors in my wheelchair, and I couldn't wheel myself because my old wheelchair was extremely heavy. I didn't feel confident asking for help, so the staff didn't escort me either—I just wanted to be "normal" and do things like the other people in my classes. I felt incredibly lonely, and this made my symptoms even worse.

After many weeks of feeling alone, I did eventually make new friends who also spent time in the learning support room. They brought me everywhere they went in the college. They helped me get my lunch, pushed my wheelchair, held doors open, came with me in the lift where we took *many* silly mirror selfies, which really cheered me up.

Finding those two people made my life a lot less lonely in college and ensured I had somebody to sit with, which I was grateful for. I contributed as much as I could to these friendships despite being very ill, and we created a good dynamic for a while—this helped me through the tough months still to come.

~

About a month into college, my health hit the worst it's ever been. These few months of my life still play on my mind, and often creep into my dreams. Being chronically ill or suffering from a neurological condition can completely turn your life upside down. It can make you feel so alone, and can make you lose hope for ever functioning again.

Medical settings can be very traumatic, and often new symptoms are scary when you're not sure what's happening or whether your symptoms are life-threatening. When you lose consciousness with episodes, the lines blur between being awake and being somewhere else—time feels like a black hole. I don't recall my specific timeline during the autumn of 2021 because my days were full of tic attacks, seizures, being paralysed, and struggling to stay conscious through lessons. That time is a whirlwind of nights in my bedroom, seizing on various floors, not knowing where I was or who people were, pain in my whole body and many more things that I often wish I could forget.

It didn't only make *my* life very distressing, but my family's too. I think it was one of the hardest times for both me and the people around me, because so much time was spent in hospitals or trying to accommodate my symptoms every single day. Constantly adapting can be incredibly draining, and it does take a toll on the people around us too.

Please look out for anybody you know who may have a chronic illness or is struggling with their health. Be kind to them and their families, and give them space to process and offer to help them when they're in need.

If you're struggling with your own health or a family member's health right now, please continue reading with caution as some scenes may be distressing—however I haven't included anything too graphic as I'd like this book to feel accessible for as many people as possible, so people can get an insight into what life with disabilities *can* look like. I want to share the story of my FND diagnosis, the hospital stays, and the hell I went through in the months where my health hit an all-time low.

Before we get stuck in, I'd like to say that since this point in my life I'm doing much, *much* better! I'm happy a lot of days, I can better manage my FND symptoms when they come along, and I've finally got answers for most of my health struggles. Leaving education—therefore having less stress in my life—has given me some happiness and *life* back, so please take this as a reminder that there are **always** ways to adapt and better suit your needs.

Due to my conditions, I could never function in a "normal" job such as waitressing or working in a shop. Mentally, I'd burn out, and physically, I'd fall into a flare-up within only a few days, meaning I'd probably be fired *and* I'd be dealing with horrific symptoms.

But, being self employed as an advocate and content creator has enabled me to make a living while organising my time in ways that suit me on the day. By watching, engaging and learning from my videos, you've all enabled me to do what I love as my job. I'm able to manage my health, accommodate for my neurodivergent brain, reduce my tics, and still do everything I love like making videos, recording music and writing this book. I'm forever thankful for everybody who leaves lovely responses and engages with my platform. It truly has changed my life.

I probably wouldn't have believed this back at the start of

college, but trust me when I say **things can get better**. There is always a light at the end of the tunnel, whether it's a big, bright spotlight or just a small flicker of candlelight. Give yourself time, be patient with yourself and do whatever you need to reduce stress. Let yourself rest.

# SEVENTEEN
# LOCKED IN MY OWN BODY

My main neurological symptoms started during my GCSE exams. These symptoms quickly became very debilitating and affected my mobility on most days. When I transitioned to college, the change triggered a huge flare-up of my conditions, as described in the last chapter.

My paralysis episodes became longer than usual—my legs didn't work for weeks on end, and I was using my wheelchair and crutches in college nearly every single day. I had more and more seizures in lessons due to the stress of concentrating, mixed with over-stimulating classroom environments. The new people, places and teachers were too much for my brain to handle, therefore my body started to shut down.

My symptoms were completely unmanaged at this time of my life, and the fast-paced, social lifestyle didn't give my brain enough time to rest and heal. This left me in a rather critical state of debilitating symptoms and constant physical and mental burnout.

There is a common overlap between neurodiversity and chronic illness, because struggling to cope with social burnout can have a *huge* effect on your physical health—this is just one reason why it's important to de-stigmatise and advocate for mental health.

~

Despite my symptoms progressively worsening for over a year and a half, I still didn't have a diagnosis or answers at the time of starting college. I'd had blood tests, scans, appointments, EEGs, and a failed MRI attempt where my tics were too violent to even get me in the machine!

Getting blood drawn can be an enormous battle when you have Tourette's. I remember after a severe cluster of seizures, I ended up in A&E with my hand completely paralysed. Doctors decided to do a blood test, which sent me into a panic because I've always had a fear of needles. These nerves quickly resulted in more tics, and the quiet hospital waiting room only made this worse. I began shouting, hitting myself, putting my middle fingers up at the other patients, until it turned into a full tic attack.

After an hour or so, the doctor called me in for the blood test and I went into a separate smaller room, still ticcing. They took one look at me and we all knew this wasn't going to be easy—I didn't think they'd actually go through with it!

After stepping out for a few minutes, the doctor came back as promised—but this time with 4 other nurses. They all crowded into the tiny room and held me down so the doctor could get the needle in my arm.

I remember feeling incredibly powerless, an this fear only fuelled my tics and made them even worse. I didn't want to hit or hurt anybody with my tics, but I was so overwhelmed by the situation that I couldn't relax.

I struggle with physical contact due to being autistic, but I couldn't express this at the time as I didn't yet have an explanation for feeling like I was about to explode.

This memory is a blur of arms, chests and pain in my arm as I twitched against the needle—it wasn't a nice experience. Unfortunately, traumatic medical experiences happen frequently to people with Tourette's, therefore having frequent medical investigations was really inconvenient alongside my tics.

If you're a doctor and you meet a patient with tics, please work through problems like this *with* your patient, letting them know each step of the way what is happening. Don't make them feel physically overwhelmed or restricted because this only makes our tics worse. Try to calm your patient down, make them feel comfortable, and ask for consent before doing any procedure or holding them down so they don't feel out of control.

My mum and I spent countless days attending appointments and following up with doctor, after doctor, *after doctor*. And yet, I still didn't have a diagnosis or the support I needed when going through the most disabling period of my life.

The NHS is incredible because it allows us to get free healthcare and support within the UK, but it definitely has faults too. People are frequently missed or pushed to the back of years-long waiting lists, leaving them to struggle without any help or treatment. People are mistreated due to the lack of staff and the stressful environments nurses have to function within, so it's becoming increasingly difficult to get the support you need.

This needs to change. People need to be supported, and they need access to the help they desperately deserve so they can live their lives with answers and treatment plans.

My FND diagnosis didn't come at the end of a waiting list as we'd expected, it actually came in the room of a stroke ward in a specialist neurology hospital.

It started as a fairly normal day for me: a few seizures, some symptoms but overall not a horrifically overwhelming or severe day. But, as usual, my symptoms worsened when evening came around. Being tired can drastically worsen my symptoms, meaning most of my severe attacks come at nighttime or after long and stressful days.

On this day, I dropped into a seizure on my bed and woke up as usual—this didn't concern me as I was used to having seizures by that point. This changed when I suddenly dropped into another seizure, falling with my face directly on my bed. I don't recall the whole seizure as I am usually unconscious, but I do remember coming around and feeling very drowsy. My head felt fuzzy, my arms felt numb and tingly with a burning pain I often struggle with, and my muscles were sore from convulsing. I had all the usual symptoms which follow a tonic-clonic seizure.

After taking a second to recover from the drowsiness, I realised something was very wrong: I couldn't move. My whole body felt like a lead weight and I couldn't even move my face. I tried to make my mouth move, but my muscles didn't let me form any words or move at all. I began to panic. I remember I couldn't even cry properly because my eyelids wouldn't move, and my chest couldn't expand enough to get more air—it was absolutely terrifying.

I found a diary entry from after this episode where I described what it feels to be completely paralysed. This may be upsetting to read, but I think it's important to share.

I want to give you a chance to understand what goes on inside somebody's head while experiencing these symptoms. Hopefully after reading this you'll have more insight into how to comfort somebody or listen to them if they need to talk about their experiences.

"I could only blink and move my eyes. I was facing the wall so I couldn't even see a clock to check the time, but I'd guess about half an hour passed and I still couldn't move anything.

I tried to speak but I couldn't say a word. I tried to shout, groan, or make any noise but nothing came out, so I just lay and panicked. The worst part was that I couldn't even physically panic because I couldn't move to cry or hyperventilate like I usually would. A few tears fell and that was the only thing that could be outwardly seen or shown. It was scary not being able to tell anybody. I hope it never happens again.

I waited, silently wishing it would go away while my whole body burned like someone was pouring fire on my legs and arms. But I still couldn't move anything or cry in reaction to what was happening. I tried so many times to say "Alexa" or "Siri" to try and call someone, but nothing would come out of my mouth. I tried to fall asleep so that time would pass because every single second was like some kind of torture, like being trapped in someone's tomb of a body and nobody hearing you."

As you can tell by reading that entry, I was scared during this episode. I didn't know what was happening and I had no way of communicating, so I lay in my bed and waited for my symptoms to improve… but they didn't go away like they usually did.

After some time, I managed to groan and make noise until my mum came into the room and helped me sit up. She propped me up onto pillows, putting one behind my head because I couldn't hold it up, and I was gradually able to move my face again. I remember feeling so thankful to be able to speak! Not having my usual methods of communication, no ways to express what was happening, and no way to ask for help was really frustrating, especially when I couldn't use pointing or signing to get my message across either.

When I re-gained verbal function, I chatted to my mum while she tested each body part for sensation, asking me if I could lift my legs or feel my toes. She said my limbs were ice cold and took photos of my purple, mottled skin to show the doctor. Mottling is where blood pools under the skin and purple rash-like marks appear, commonly seen when you're very cold or in people who don't have great circulation.

If I tried to move a part of my body that was paralysed, it was like shouting when the communication lines were down. Like shouting into a phone when the battery has died. My body couldn't "hear" my brain or receive any of the signals.

I thought with all the power in my brain, *"legs you need to move, lift up!"* but they'd stay completely still. I'd experienced this before in my legs, but this time the feeling was in my whole body including my neck, meaning I couldn't even turn my head or lift it up to look at something.

After a while, I was *very* bored because I couldn't do *anything* to entertain myself; I had to sit and stare at the same wall in my bedroom. My mum rang my best friend so I could chat to him while she went and made some food, placing my phone on my bedside table so we could chat on FaceTime.

When I recently asked him about this day, he said "I remember speaking to you on a call while your mum fed you cheese on toast like a pigeon feeding a baby pigeon" which made me laugh! I'd forgotten how much he cheered me up during that scary episode, and I'm always grateful for jokes and laughter from the people I love.

In my usual positive spirits, I managed to stay upbeat and laughing after I'd calmed down from the initial panic. People often describe me as a smiley person because I try to focus on the positive or funny parts of situations, otherwise I'd feel really sad. Being autistic, I experience emotions very deeply, so telling light-hearted jokes or focusing on "glimmers" and happy moments is definitely a coping mechanism I default to.

My mum recorded this episode for my doctors, and I also asked her to document feeding me the cheese on toast, because it was a light-hearted moment which gave a glimpse into how debilitating my symptoms can be. It was such a bizarre night, and I'd never want anybody else to experience having no sensation or movement in their whole body—it felt somewhat dehumanising and extremely uncomfortable.

After five or six hours I was still completely paralysed from the neck down and my mum became concerned because my symptoms didn't usually last this long. We didn't know that my symptoms *were* FND at this point—though we'd heard of and researched the condition thanks to people mentioning it to me online.

We ended up calling 999 for an ambulance but had to wait over two hours. Covid lockdowns meant the NHS was struggling immensely. Some people had to wait over twelve hours for ambulances, therefore we were actually lucky to only wait for two hours. When the paramedics came, I had no improvement in mobility so they took all of my vitals. My blood sugar was really low, so they fed me a sachet of really gross glucose gel to bring my sugar levels back up. It tasted absolutely awful, but it did make my levels improve, so hurray for the strange-flavoured sachet I guess!

After taking note of all my symptoms and checking me over, the paramedics weren't sure where to send me. My symptoms aligned with some dangerous neurological possibilities—they thought I could be having a stroke!

Even after explaining that I'd experienced similar symptoms before, they put me on the stroke pathway and sent me in an ambulance to a specialist neurology hospital. I was alone with the paramedic in the ambulance and I remember trying to look at all the signs and medical equipment to distract myself (plus, I'm very nosy), however I still couldn't move my head properly so this was rather difficult. On the drive to the hospital, I had a few smaller seizures which involved no movement or convulsions—my body wasn't receiving any signals and still couldn't move, even during my seizures.

This was my first time being in an adult hospital ward. I was sixteen at the time, so it was strange being the youngest person there, especially as most of the stroke patients in the department were elderly.

They took my blood and placed a cannula (a little tube inserted into your arm to give quick access to your bloodstream) in case I had another seizure and they needed to give me medication. This was probably the easiest needle experience I've ever had, since I couldn't move or tic my body at all! All of the mental fear was still there, but I physically couldn't pull away or twitch.

A few different doctors checked me out until I was eventually placed in a corridor to wait until morning. My mum and I had to sit (well, technically I was lying down) on a stretcher in the corridor for the whole night because there weren't enough rooms to give every patient a proper bed. This is unfortunately very common here in the UK, but at least I *did* get seen by doctors!

TW - Be careful reading this chapter if you suffer with medical trauma, PTSD or with topics surrounding death, blood, or hospital emergencies.

I have a vivid memory of watching the nurses walk past, when suddenly a beeping alarm blared out from nearby. I knew this was a "code blue" alarm from TV shows where somebody's heart stops beating and the monitors begin to beep continuously.

I saw doctors wheeling a trolley carrying a man who was covered in blood. He was intubated, meaning he had a tube placed in his throat so the doctors could use a bag to breathe for him, and they were also performing CPR. It was absolute chaos. I remember watching the scene unfold and not being able to look away because I couldn't move—I watched as they wheeled the man past me and took him to another part of the hospital.

I felt shaken; I'd never seen somebody in such a critical state before, and I wished I could have turned my head the other way to compose myself. I don't know if the man was okay, but I really hope he made it out in the end and survived.

I wanted to share that memory because it shaped the way I think about hospitals now. Seeing somebody flatline and be wheeled past me really highlighted how fragile our lives are, and how many people have to witness similar scenarios every day.

So many disabled or chronically ill people are exposed to heartbreaking or difficult situations due to the amount of time they spend in hospitals or with other severely ill people. This can lead to people developing medical trauma.

It's not something that's talked about very much, but it's a harsh reality for a lot of people. My experiences are only one case in the millions of people who suffer traumatic events or treatment within hospitals, so if you know anybody who has been through medical treatment or a family member has become sick, then please try to support them and let them know that you are there if they need anything.

Don't invalidate people's experiences, and try to understand that medical treatments, tests, or difficult symptoms can leave a lasting effect on people, even if they don't seem traumatic to you from the outside. Be kind and sensitive when talking to people about what they've been through, and make sure to ask for consent before you bring up memories which could be difficult or triggering for people to talk about.

Personally, I enjoy sharing my story and telling people about my conditions because I want to help other people feel seen. I hope to educate those who haven't experienced disability before. But, not everybody likes to talk about their medical history. Not all of us like to openly or publicly acknowledge that we're disabled, and that's okay!

Every experience is different, and every person is affected by their experiences in different ways to others, so something that seems "fine" to one person might have been very traumatic to somebody else.

～

Finally… after many hours of waiting, my movement started to return! At the ten-hour mark of being paralysed, the feeling returned in my neck and I could gradually move my shoulders, arms, and hands again. I could finally use my phone, drink water by myself, and look around the room freely. My legs however, stayed paralysed for much longer and took weeks to properly function again.

When morning came, the neurologist did a full body neuro-logical exam which obviously showed a lack of movement in my legs. I showed her the videos of my various symptoms and gave her all the information we'd shown to previous doctors. After a long discussion, more exams from another neurologist, and her consulting with other doctors… I was diagnosed with Functional Neurological Disorder.

I finally had answers! She told me that all the symptoms I'd been experiencing were due to FND and reassured my mum that my seizures weren't epileptic, therefore were not causing direct damage to my brain. This was an enormous relief because it's dangerous for epileptic seizures to go on longer than five minutes because this can lead to brain damage and in severe cases, even death. But, because my seizures were non-epileptic, we didn't have to worry as much about my seizures—aside from the obvious dangers of falling or injuring myself.

A couple of months later—when I was more recovered and walking again—we had another appointment with an FND specialist; this was one of the most *validating* medical experiences I've had!

The doctor knew so much about FND; he nodded whenever I told him something I struggled with (because he'd actually heard of it, and knew why it was happening!) and he explained everything about the condition that I needed to know in order to live more happily. He suggested lifestyle changes like stress reduction and avoiding events to help reduce flare-ups, and he told me that my symptoms *could* and *would* improve if I took care of myself well, acknowledged my symptoms and accepted them so I could learn to live *with* them rather than fighting them. This positively altered my mindset so that I always try to adapt my surroundings, accommodating for my needs so I can live more freely even when my symptoms are there.

Don't worry if you're not at this stage in your acceptance and understanding journey yet: it's a long process. I'm fairly flexible in adapting to new diagnoses due to my previous experience developing Tourette's, so I like to think I handled my FND pretty well.

I also had the privilege of finding a doctor who believed and listened to me, teaching my family how to cope with my condition. Not everybody has access to healthcare, and if I hadn't been rushed to hospital that night, I don't think I'd have been diagnosed for much, *much* longer.

Waiting lists are too long and hospitals are constantly full. Specialists are few and far between, meaning so many people (like those of you reading this who are undergoing investigations right now) are left without answers or even an appointment to get seen.

It's okay to feel disheartened; I know it feels beyond frustrating when you're not listened to or validated. Remember that you *can* research your symptoms and find resources online even before you have confirmation of diagnosis, but I don't advise taking any treatments or making changes without the advice of a trained medical professional. Clinical diagnosis are extremely important, especially when it comes to treatment or medication, because the wrong treatment—or lack of treatment—can be really harmful.

But, it's worth recognising that there is a whole mental battle when developing a chronic illness or disability too, and this isn't always defined by a medical diagnosis.

You can begin your acceptance journey by accepting the presence of your symptoms and learning how you can cope with them. Whether it's FND, mental illness, physical disability, chronic illness or something else, try to be patient with yourself and allow any emotions to flow which are needed to grieve your non-disabled life. This is a process a large proportion of disabled people unfortunately have to go through.

You will come to understand your condition and your needs better as time goes on, and you will move up those waiting lists (even if it's slowly) and one day you'll finally receive the medical attention you need and deserve. I sincerely hope this is soon for those of you who need it.

# EIGHTEEN
## GETTING ANSWERS

Alongside my Tourette's, I finally had my diagnosis of FND. This stands for Functional Neurological Disorder, which affects how the nervous system works and how the signals between the brain and the body are sent and received. This can cause malfunctioning in parts of the body or systems within the brain, which causes a wide plethora of symptoms. Having FND can make it extremely difficult for us to function or do daily tasks.

Symptoms of FND can include:

- Non-epileptic seizures (also known as NEAD)
- Limb weakness or paralysis
- Tremors
- Sudden twitching or muscle jerking (myoclonic jerks)
- Limb dystonia (involuntary muscle contractions which cause abnormal postures)
- Spasms and contractures (where tendons become fixed in awkward or uncomfortable positions)
- Problems with walking motions (gait), posture, or balance

- Drop attacks or sleep attacks
- Muscle stiffness
- Tics

Other symptoms affecting brain function can also include:

- Speech difficulties (eg. sudden onset of stuttering)
- Problems with seeing or hearing (sensory impairments)
- Pain (including chronic migraines)
- Extreme slowness and fatigue
- Numbness or inability to sense touch
- Memory loss
- Difficulty concentrating

These symptoms may have a sudden onset or they may increase gradually over time. Severity or frequency may increase when attention is drawn to symptoms, and may decrease when the person is distracted. For some people, FND symptoms can go away! However, in other cases, FND symptoms may last for years and become very debilitating, hindering people's quality of life significantly.

FND is a widely misunderstood condition which medical professionals still don't fully understand due to not enough research being funded. This means there isn't a lot of post-diagnostic help available for people with FND. There is no known cure and there aren't any specific treatments or medications available to help, which leaves us feeling pretty helpless or "in the dark" about our own condition.

FND is commonly known as a "software" problem which means the dysfunction lies in the sending and receiving of signals in the brain (the "software"), rather than damage to the physical structure of the brain (the "hardware" in this analogy).

This means that someone with FND *can* technically function normally, but they can't when their symptoms appear due to a disconnection in the functioning of our brains with the rest of our body.

NES (non-epileptic seizures) or NEAD (non-epileptic attack disorder) can be worsened by stress, emotions, or can sometimes develop after traumatic events, although this definitely isn't always the case. Seizures in FND are most common in women (or AFAB people) and often begin in young adulthood. Episodes may become very frequent and prolonged, and in my case lasted up to forty minutes with multiple seizures happening in a row—this is known as a seizure cluster.

No single test can confirm a diagnosis of FND. A neurologist and psychologists usually work together to look for specific patterns of signs and symptoms to reach a diagnosis. They may also run tests such as physical, neurological, and psychiatric exams, as well as imaging scans, which are often used to rule out other causes and investigate symptoms such as tremors, weakness, walking, and vision differences.

My FND diagnosis involved a few tests like multiple EEGs, blood tests, ECGs and more. It's often a long and frustrating journey to get answers for neurological symptoms, and I definitely felt disheartened many times in my own diagnostic process. It can feel like nobody truly understands what is going on, and some doctors don't listen to us at all. Chronic illness patients are too-often blamed for our symptoms, being told we're "fine" and being passed around different departments when no doctors can get to the bottom of our symptoms.

Many doctors aren't trained in complex chronic conditions or functional disorders like FND because research has only properly progressed in recent years. Some doctors don't believe symptoms are real when they can't find an immediate or visible cause, leaving many people with no help or support, no diagnosis, and a boat-load of isolating self-doubt due to being told we're making it all up.

This happens to so many disabled people when it shouldn't be happening at all—doctors should investigate people's symptoms and treat them with respect and kindness, without belittling them or making them feel like they don't fit into the "correct" boxes.

If you're in a similar process to this, please know that it is not your fault if doctors struggle to find a cause for your symptoms. You are not a burden, you *do* deserve answers. With time and the right doctors, those answers *will* be out there.

One of the main tests used to investigate seizures is an EEG (or electroencephalogram) which is usually performed to detect epileptic brain activity. This involves sticking many wires (electrodes) to the scalp and other points on the body to monitor brainwaves. Doctors may attempt to trigger an episode by using flashing lights or rapid breathing tests because these are common triggers for seizures.

EEGs are useful for epileptic patients, but scans often come back as clear for patients with FND. This does *not* mean that we aren't experiencing symptoms or that the seizures aren't real, it just shows that they aren't *epileptic*—this is not a reason for doctors to invalidate patients!

Studies show that FND can be caused by trauma, head injuries, a response to stress, or in some cases have no known trigger at all. This has proven that FND is not purely psychological, contrary to the misconception coined by Freud's theory of Conversion Disorder in 1894.

Anybody can develop Functional Neurological Disorder—about 4 to 12 people per 100,000 will develop FND and biological factors can make someone more susceptible. The condition may develop as a result of an illness, physical trauma, an operation or life event. Other triggers may include childhood trauma, early life stress, long-term anxiety, abuse or even interpersonal relationships. FND is commonly experienced alongside anxiety, depression, PTSD, other neurological conditions like Tourette's, or chronic illnesses such as Fibromyalgia, however people can still develop symptoms without any psychological factors.

FND is labelled as a neuropsychiatric condition, meaning it is a disorder that sits in between the fields of neurology and psychiatry; both biological and psychological factors can play a role in making people more likely to develop the condition. FND links with psychiatry when triggers or stressors stem from past or present emotional trauma—in these cases, therapies such as trauma therapy, CBT, EMDR or counselling can sometimes help manage people's mental health, which could aid in reducing their physical symptoms. But, it's important to note that therapy doesn't suit everybody's needs, and in most cases, you can't cure chronic illnesses by simply prioritising mental well-being.

Sometimes a diagnosis of FND is mistakenly given to patients who have an underlying condition with similar symptoms—such as PANS or PANDAS—because these autoimmune conditions aren't yet widely known or even recognised by the NHS (the UK's healthcare system).

An FND diagnosis should only be given when you have the clinical features of the condition, and not only because there's minimal evidence of alternative conditions. Where you can, try to advocate for yourself and reach out to relevant communities or charities, as they can aid you in locating neurologists, recommending treatments, or finding adaptations to try.

The root cause of FND is still unknown. It has been misunderstood for many years, and misconceptions surrounding the condition are unfortunately very common. Despite onset being triggered by psychological factors in some cases, FND is a very physical disorder which affects mobility, limb function, brain function, bladder or bowel function, cognitive function and so much more. It can severely affect our quality of life.

It is important to remember that FND is not a mental health disorder; it is a neurological condition. We don't have control over our symptoms—they are physically disabling and often painful. Developing FND is not a choice.

If you have FND, it is essential to remember that your symptoms are REAL! Nobody should gaslight you, or insinuate that you are imagining things. If medical tests don't draw visible conclusions, please know that you are *still* valid and there are so many other people in the community who are experiencing similar scenarios. In the UK, there are charities such as *FND Hope UK* where you can find support, along with different Facebook groups or meetups where you can connect with others like you.

～

My diagnosis experience was traumatic at first, but when I finally received official confirmation and explanations for my symptoms, it felt like my entire world had been explained. I felt heard, understood, and I finally felt seen. My neurologist explained how my symptoms worked and that I wasn't alone, he told me ways I could learn to manage the condition, gave me tips and suggested aids I could use to help get me through flare-ups. I finally felt validated.

My FND has been debilitating for many years now, and although my current lifestyle manages and accommodates my health much better than before, I still have debilitating symptoms. I've been forced to completely change the way I live, learning to plan my life in a way which accommodates my symptoms. I have to very carefully plan trips and events, avoid stressful social occasions, avoid friendship groups due to the amount of stress this causes, and I've had to live a much slower and more intentional life just to stay afloat. Surprisingly, I've slowly learned that I do actually prefer a slow lifestyle, as this reduces my FND symptoms, lessens my tics, and also limits social stress for me as an autistic person.

FND is not an easy-to-manage or curable condition, but there are ways to live a happy life even with the condition. I will probably have FND for the rest of my life, however I may not have the same symptoms for the whole time. Flare-ups will likely come and go along with stress levels and different phases in my life.

Like with my Tourette's diagnosis, it was difficult to accept I had FND because I knew there wasn't a magic pill to make it go away. There weren't any treatments to "fix" my brain, and there wasn't a definitive way to make me "better". My family found the long-term concept difficult to accept too. Even though we were relieved to have answers, it was hard hearing confirmation that I had such an unheard-of and difficult to manage condition.

I've now accepted that I have FND, and I'm okay with it. My symptoms can definitely be awful to experience, and I often wish they could disappear… but I've become a lot more resilient and my perspective on the world has actually changed! I recognise more things to be grateful for, and I will never take advantage of being able to do things again. If I wake up and my legs work, I'm immediately grateful because I know what it feels like to have that taken away. If I go a day or a week without a seizure, I'm thankful because I've experienced weeks where I don't even remember my own name due to being unconscious so frequently.

I've learned to slow down, stop and appreciate the tiny things in life: the glimmers. I look up at the sky every day and admire all the clouds I can see. I listen to the birds, the rain and the animals in the forest. I enjoy every moment I can with the people around me, simply because I'm able to.

If you're having a difficult time, look around you and find one thing you can appreciate the beauty of. Perhaps it's your bedroom, your decor, or a pet you have. Does it make you smile? Do you have a cosy blanket that you love the texture of? Maybe you can see the sun out of your window, and you can feel thankful for the nice weather. Maybe you have a sibling or a parent nearby who you can appreciate for being in your life. Have they helped you and loved you? Do you have friends who take on this role in your life instead? Can you simply appreciate that *you* are here for you?

There is *always* a reason to appreciate the world and feel thankful for existing—even when everything feels like it's falling down. I've found this perspective to help me so much, because if I focus on the negative side of my situation, I only become more sad and frustrated that I have to live like this. Yes, it's annoying that I can't be "normal" or do things as easily as I used to, and there are days when I cry and just wish that life could've dealt me an easier hand.

But, I refuse to throw away all the possible good memories by wishing I was different. I refuse to spend any more of my precious time wishing I could magically be somebody else, or that I could undo events of the past. The only thing we can do right now is to exist and be here right now. We can choose to be present and simply exist in whatever state or stage of life we're currently in, and I find it helpful to stop and acknowledge this—maybe you'll find this helpful too.

If you've recently received a diagnosis—or perhaps you're struggling to process an old one—then try to give yourself some space to just *be*. You are living, you are here, you are trying, and that alone is amazing. No matter how much your life has changed, there *are* things you can do and there *are* so many reasons to be proud of yourself.

You can be disabled and still be a vital part of a community. You can still travel and enjoy the world if you plan accordingly and put accommodations in place. You can find hobbies you enjoy, even if you need an adapted version or the help of a physiotherapist or instructor.

You are so capable, so please don't let yourself feel like your diagnosis or disability makes you any less worthy.

# NINETEEN
# APPOINTMENT ADVICE

I want to give you a few tips I've learned from over seven years of attending medical appointments and finding communication methods to help me make the most out of appointments. This is especially helpful if you're going through a diagnostic process for example, but I've included more generalised bullet points which can be applied to any type of appointment.

Hopefully this list will give you some ideas for how to accommodate yourself—whether you're neurodivergent, if this is your first appointment, or even if you're a long-term patient, there are always new tips to learn!

## HOW CAN YOU PLAN FOR APPOINTMENTS?

- **Prepare** by making **symptom lists** of anything you've been experiencing.
- Bring a list of all medications and **past medical history** or medical files you have. You may want to include past experiences, mental health struggles, and any recent life changes, but make sure to mention what is most relevant to your specific appointment.

- Bring a **notepad** or your phone to take notes. It can be difficult to recall what the doctor has said, so I highly suggest taking notes or asking for a written follow-up so you can process the information at a later time.
- Prepare a **list of questions** before the appointment to make sure you cover everything that's needed with your doctor. Those minutes are precious, so make sure you cover everything you intended to make sure you get the most out of the visit as possible.
- Be as **honest and open** with your doctor as you can, because this gives them the most accurate portrayal of your symptoms. Don't play down your pain or your symptoms, though I know this is habit for many of us with long-term conditions.
- Speak with your doctor about **resources and support groups** for you and your family post-diagnosis.
- If you can, **bring a family member** or friend for support so they can help remember anything the doctor said. Appointments can be very overwhelming and if you're like me, then you forget *everything* once you leave the room! This friend or family member can also advocate for you if you struggle to navigate social settings or speak during appointments, which can help to minimise any patronising attitudes or mistreatment towards patients (especially neurodivergent or autistic people).
- Work with your friends, family, doctors or care team to **set goals,** whether it's a new treatment plan, new medication, a referral to a specific department or even asking for a specific test to help diagnose your symptoms.
- Trying **lifestyle changes** such as doing physiotherapy or exercise, eating foods which are good for you, reducing stress (this may include meditation or doing hobbies you enjoy), and getting enough sleep.

Reducing your anxiety or mental stress can sometimes improve symptoms, especially with conditions like FND.

- If you have physically visible symptoms (for example, seizures, paralysis or tics), I'd suggest **filming episodes** when they happen so that you have videos to show during appointments. I sent all of my symptom videos to my doctors after they requested I start documenting my episodes; this was incredibly helpful in diagnosing and identifying my seizures!

There are of course *many* other resources and strategies which can help you during assessments or appointments, but this is how I personally prepare for any check-ups, phone calls, or in-person appointments.

I know waiting for answers can be difficult, so here are some reminders for anybody struggling with diagnosis, appointments, mental health, a disability, or anybody who needs reassurance that you are valid and that you are worthy and deserving of support.

## REMINDERS:

- No matter how much doctors patronise or dismiss you, please know that your symptoms are *not* your fault.
- You should not have to advocate for yourself in order to be worthy of being listened to. You should be listened to and accommodated for even with communication difficulties.
- Your diagnosis—whether you've received one yet or not—does not define you! It may change your

perspective or change your life, but you are *always* a person before you are a condition.

- You are loved, and developing a disability does not change this. The people who truly deserve you will stay, and anybody who judges or sees you differently is not worth your energy! Trust me, you're better off without them. Please try to let any negative people go so that you can move forward and *live*.

- You can be happy and live a full life. It doesn't matter if you're disabled, or if you struggle with mobility, energy, mental or physical restrictions, there are ways you can accommodate, medications to take, adaptations to put in place, and people to surround you who can make your life shine brightly again.

- You don't have to be "fixed" to be worthy of enjoying life. Being disabled does not mean we can't have fun or laugh and enjoy things again, it just means we have to work slightly differently!

- It is *okay* not to do the same things as non-disabled people, and needing to rest or saying no to things does not make you any less valuable.

- You shouldn't be ashamed to show your disability, because nobody should make you feel embarrassed or like you're unwelcome. The world can be cruel sometimes, but know that this is not a reflection of you. You do not need to change or hide in order to appear more "worthy" or like less of a burden.

I welcome you to be the brightest (or darkest, technically it's up to you) person you can be. Wear the most vibrant clothing you can find no matter how much you stand out, unmask any stims or behaviours you feel "childish" for, let your tics out freely, sing, dance, and just be YOU!

You are unique and that is the most special thing in the world. You *are* enough, just as you are.

# TWENTY
# LEARNING TO WALK AGAIN

Although I gained some mobility back after my FND diagnosis, my legs stayed paralysed for a while longer. Chronic illness or neurological flare-ups are often unpredictable and can vary in length or severity.

During the autumn I started college, I experienced the worst flare up I've ever had. I couldn't walk for months and I was frequently stuck in my bedroom due to my house and lifestyle being inaccessible. Luckily, my college had lifts, so (unlike secondary school) I could still attend classes when using my wheelchair—but this doesn't mean I was *well* enough to actually complete the work.

My physical mobility slowly improved over the next few months, but my mental health was rapidly declining. My seizures, brain fog, memory loss, confusion, sensory issues and many other symptoms became so debilitating that I struggled to stay awake during the day. I couldn't focus or even fathom sitting through lessons and completing a full college day. My body physically hurt, and I often had severe headaches and drowsiness from all the seizure episodes and fainting. I struggled to even engage with my friends.

This foggy feeling did slowly improve over time, and after

finally getting a diagnosis—therefore having answers to why this was happening—meant that I could adapt parts of my life to help reduce symptoms.

After taking a week off college post-diagnosis, my mum immediately set up a meeting with support staff from my college's disability department. The staff were always willing to take me to lessons, walk (or wheel) me to my mum's car, and they sat with me through more episodes than I could count. One of the learning support staff, Kylie, supported me for the whole two years I went to college and never failed to cheer me up, no matter how debilitating my symptoms were at the time.

While on the topic of college, I want to share that I seriously considered giving up during that first term (the autumn months) of college: one of my options was dropping out.

Despite having adaptions, speaking to support staff about dropping subjects, cutting my schedule down, and working from home instead of attending classes in person, I thought I wouldn't make it through.

We cut out all of my form classes and registration, RE (religious education) and any extracurriculars or assemblies that were usually mandatory—this left me with only my three main subjects to attend. We set up online learning via Teams so I could log on to my lessons online when I wasn't physically well enough to attend in person. This was incredibly helpful and one of the main reasons I managed to keep up!

I highly recommend asking your school or college to consider this accommodation if you feel it would benefit you, because most schools already incorporated online learning during the Covid period, so I strongly believe this should be offered as a continued option for those of us with disabilities.

As the weeks went by, I fell into a routine of doing half of my lessons in-person and half via Microsoft Teams. I also caught up on missed lessons at home, which gave me the ability to rest and focus on my health a little more. My FND symptoms finally lessened once I adapted my routine and reduced the immense levels of stress I'd been under.

Recovery from FND flare-ups can take weeks or even months, and sometimes there are cases where people's symptoms are permanent. Please keep this in mind when seeing content by disabled creators, or when encountering people with FND because we all have different needs. No two people are the same, and no two flare-ups are the same either.

It took around two months for the use of my legs to fully come back, and I had to do physio exercises every day to gradually improve my mobility. I saw an occupational therapist who helped to secure a few adaptations in my house like grab bars in our bathroom, a bath-board so I could shower sitting down, and also a second banister for our stairs for safer holding.

The sensations in my legs came back first, then I gained some small movement and was eventually was able to bear weight again. I looked like Bambi on ice for the first few weeks! Thankfully, my legs did go back to normal, and by 2022 I was finally doing able to do the things I loved again.

During this period, I had to face a lot of internalised ableism and stigma surrounding independence and disability. Even though I'd had Tourette's for a few years before my FND diagnosis, this was a *whole* new plethora of symptoms, new realities, and a different set of needs to accept.

I often needed help to get to the bathroom and I couldn't dress myself when I had symptoms in my hands. If I had an arm paralysed or locked up then I needed help to shower, wash my hair, and also feed myself. I remember being fed by friends in both secondary school and college while my arms no longer worked—this was a jarring concept to accept, and it made me feel like a baby or like I was inadequate or incapable, even though I'd never think this about anybody else who needed support.

There is *nothing* wrong with needing help or having to ask for accommodations, even if they feel embarrassing. It's so hard to accept suddenly needing help with basic tasks like washing yourself or getting out of bed, but it is **not** your fault. You are no less of a person because you can't function quite the same as somebody who isn't disabled.

Needing physical help due to a disability as a teenager can feel like the "worst" thing in the world. I lost all sense of inde-pendence, my privacy, and a lot of dignity as I suddenly needed help with more personal tasks like showering and changing. But, after dealing with my own insecurities and doing lots of inner work, I am not ashamed of needing help, and I don't think it should be embarrassing to talk about.

Who decided that needing adaptations or help to get dressed is embarrassing? Whoever decided needing a carer is a taboo topic? Who decided we shouldn't talk about these things or risk being judged?

I want to claim this part of my disabled life back and show that it is *not* embarrassing or shameful to need help. Being assisted in public shouldn't frowned upon. Being fed by some-body when out for a meal shouldn't invite people to stare or patronise you. It shouldn't be socially unacceptable to talk about experiences as a disabled person, because this is just our reality! It may look different to other people's reality, but every human is unique and we all need different adaptations to help us get through life. This diversity should not only be accepted, but uplifted.

~

I've already mentioned some disability aids I use to manage my symptoms, but I'd like to share all the resources which have helped my tics and FND symptoms. I hope this can reassure you about needing adaptations for your conditions too.

You are never "too young" to be disabled and there is no "qualification" or "criteria" for you to meet in order to use a disability aid (provided it is safe for you to do so). I cannot stress enough that if it would improve your life and make things easier for you, use the aid! Use or wear it proudly, because you deserve to get through your day in the easiest or most pain-free way possible.

A helpful mindset I've come across which has helped me validate my own needs is that if you were able-bodied and completely healthy, using something like a walking stick or wheelchair wouldn't even cross your mind—you'd simply walk and think nothing of it.

Disclaimer - this next section is not medical advice and I am not a doctor, this is a list put together from my own research and lived experience as a disabled person. You should always consult your doctor before changing anything such as medication or treatment plans.

## USEFUL ADAPTATIONS AND DISABILITY AIDS:

**Hot water bottles, heat packs and cold packs.**
I struggle to think of any conditions which wouldn't benefit from some form of temperature regulation, but some examples are: using heat to relax sore muscles from tics or to help with cramps or muscle pains, soothing headaches or joint pain, easing period pains or PCOS (Polycystic Ovary Syndrome) pain, using ice packs to cool down during a POTS episode, and so much more. Similarly, ice packs can help to reduce swelling after tic

attacks or any joint injuries due to hypermobility, EDS (Ehlers-Danlos Syndrome), or from falls.

**Splints, braces, wraps and joint tape.**
These can be especially helpful for people with hypermobility or chronic illnesses such as EDS or HSD, but many people may benefit from joint support. I use braces to support tic injuries and during FND dystonia episodes where my limbs lock in strange positions. Splints are more rigid and have a metal panel down the middle, so these are ideal for keeping my wrists or ankles straight when dystonia kicks in. Padded wraps can help protect my joints when I have violent tics, and can prevent injuries when I'm repetitively ticcing one joint or hitting parts of my body.

**Compression socks or stockings.**
For people with orthostatic intolerance or POTS (Postural Orthostatic Tachycardia Syndrome), using compression socks can improve circulation and help relieve dizziness and pre-syncope symptoms. For me, wearing compression socks means that I can stand up without passing out and I often feel much less fatigued on days where I have my compression socks on. I highly recommend these!

**Portable toilets or a bedpan.**
This can be difficult and confronting to buy for the first time, but getting a bedpan can be useful for those suffering from things like chronic fatigue, severe ME/CFS, debilitating mobility problems, or paralysis. If you're unable to walk to your bathroom, then please make sure you have a safe way to manage your needs because we all need to pee! There's often a lot of stigma that toilet aids are only used by elderly people or in

hospitals, but bed pans (or "chamber pots" if we're going old-school) are used by many disabled people to prevent worsening their symptoms by moving to the bathroom when they're physically unwell.


**Seeing an occupational therapist.**

An OT can offer appropriate accommodations for your house to help with any mobility limitations (the NHS can provide home assessments in the UK). This could be a stair lift, adding a bath lift or walk-in shower, grab rails to pull yourself out of the bath or help you up from seating, widened doorways, lowering kitchen worktops, building outdoor ramps, a step rail and much more.

My family's house is quite inaccessible. We have two floors with lots of steps and we can't easily change this to make using a wheelchair easier, but there are still a few adaptations we put in place. OT installed grab rails, a second banister, and also small adaptations like a rubber circle in the kitchen to help open bottles or jars when I have weak hands. I have crutches to help me get around inside my house, because I can't use my wheelchair due to stairs.

Even with challenges and limitations, there are always small hacks or changes you can put in place to make your home more accessible for you.


**Using different mobility aids.**

Whether it's crutches, a walking stick, or any other type of mobility aid, these can all help with balance, standing and walking. I know an immense amount of people who use crutches and walking sticks on a daily basis! These tools are readily available, and they can prolong the time people with chronic illnesses can stand for, which ultimately enables us to do more in a day without flaring up.

Portable, folding crutches are perfect for travelling or taking in a backpack for a day trip. My friend Neve first showed me these back in 2021, and it blew me away how handy they were!

**Using a wheelchair.**

My wheelchairs bring me so much freedom when my body can't hold me up. They've allowed me to go out shopping, explore the world, and spend time in the fresh air when my symptoms are debilitating—this freedom changed my entire perspective to living *with* my conditions rather than constantly wishing to get rid of them.

It's important to note that you don't have to be permanently paralysed or have a physical disfigurement to warrant 'needing' a wheelchair. There are many reasons somebody may use a wheelchair, and many ambulatory wheelchair users (like me) use mobility aids to conserve energy, manage symptoms, and prevent pain or fatigue crashes. Not all wheelchair users are paralysed!

~

I bought my first ever wheelchair during secondary school, but I purchased my second (and current) wheelchair after my big health flare-up at the start of college. At first, I had a standard hospital size wheelchair with high armrests on both sides and no seat cushion. It was very heavy and rarely fit through doorways, meaning I couldn't access a lot of places. I also couldn't push the wheels by myself further than a few metres, therefore had to be pushed by friends or family most of the time.

We soon realised it was time to invest in a custom wheelchair —one which would fit my exact width and have a much lighter frame and wheels. This pricey investment was terrifying at first, but I am incredibly glad I bit the bullet and splurged on a new chair because it has *changed* my life!

The word choice "splurged" indicates a lot of money, and I'm here to tell you that custom wheelchairs are damn expensive. They range from around £800 in some brands to well over £10,000 in others. I'd put a few hundred pounds aside for a chair, but seeing the price tags at wheelchair showrooms was overwhelming.

You may wonder why I didn't just get a chair on the NHS, and trust me, I wish I could've! I first assumed I could apply for a chair and at least receive *some* help, but waiting lists are far too long and even then, help isn't guaranteed unless you use a wheelchair full-time or are deemed a priority case—the system is often not inclusive of chronic illness patients or ambulatory wheelchair users.

After searching online for different chairs, I luckily found a second-hand chair which was my exact measurements. From the moment I saw the listing, I knew this chair was *ideal*—but it was well out of my budget.

I shared my dilemma online and a viewer suggested I create a fundraiser for the new wheelchair. This felt uncomfortable at first because I didn't want to ask strangers on the internet for money. It felt wrong when people *already* supported me through comments and messages, but I finally decided that if people were asking to help and wanted to chip in, then maybe it's okay to let them. I set up a fundraiser which raised over a thousand pounds! This money paid off a large chunk of my wheelchair, meaning I could finally get one to suit my needs.

Before I continue, I want to say a massive, humongous, bigger-than-you-can-imagine THANK YOU to everybody who helped, shared and donated at the time. You gave me the gift of a custom mobility aid and changed my life during an incredibly tough part of my journey. My wheelchair still changes and improves my life to this day. I'll never be able to repay every single person who contributed, but I hope that writing this book and sharing content every day can spread awareness for disabilities and somewhat repay the favour to those people out there. You are so kind.

After bidding on the chair, I nervously waited for the auction to end. My heart was pumping through my chest. As the listing finally finished, a message popped up and told me that I'd lost the bid. I didn't get the chair, and had been outbid at the very last second. My heart sank and my eyes welled up with tears instantly.

I showed the notification to my mum and she felt sad too, but when I looked across the living room at my step-dad, his face slowly turned into a smile. He turned his phone screen around and showed me an order confirmation. He'd got the chair! The wheelchair was mine and it would arrive in less than a week.

When my new wheelchair arrived, it was drastically different from my old one. I now have a Tiga Sub 4 from RGK Wheelchairs. The frame weighs only four kilograms (yes, really!) and the wheels easily slide on and off with the click of a button. The back is lower to allow more range of motion and also folds down so it's more compact when travelling. I have foldable push handles to limit when people can push me or not, and there's a handy little pouch on the back where I can put my phone and keys.

I've recently decorated the spokes of my wheels with rainbow covers so my wheels are colourful, expressing my personality as well as helping me move around. I highly suggest adding some personality to your mobility aids, because it can make it feel like *yours* rather than looking clinical. Making your wheelchair feel "cool" or colourful can assist your acceptance and confidence journey, so do whatever you need to do in order to feel more confident in yourself!

If you aren't a wheelchair user yourself, I hope this begins to reframe your attitude towards mobility aids. Wheelchairs aren't something we need to feel bad or sorry about, and most people who use them are often grateful to have access to such a useful aid. No, it isn't nice that we're disabled and *need* to use one, but the aid itself is a brilliant tool!

Try not to be sympathetic to people purely because they're in a wheelchair. We're simply living our lives just like you are, so we don't need any apologies or prayers when we're trying to do our weekly shopping. This is worth keeping in mind when interacting with wheelchair users—treat us just as you would anybody else.

# TWENTY-ONE
# DYSAUTONOMIA

The word dysautonomia is an umbrella term for conditions relating to the disruption of the autonomic nervous system (also known as the ANS). The ANS manages all the bodily processes you don't think about—this includes blood pressure, body temperature, breathing, digestion, heart rate, sweating and more. This may sound complicated, but before freaking out at the scientific language, it's actually more simple than it sounds!

The type of dysautonomia or autonomic dysfunction that I suffer with is called **orthostatic intolerance**, which means my blood doesn't circulate (pump) around my body fast enough. This causes a lot of symptoms like dizziness, blood pooling in my limbs, vision blacking out, and fainting.

These symptoms present similarly to conditions like POTS (Postural Orthostatic Tachycardia Syndrome) which my doctors are currently investigating. This is a condition which is characterised by orthostatic intolerance and is caused by an abnormal response of the autonomic nervous system (ANS). Symptoms include (but are not limited to) increased heart-rate upon standing, dizziness, fatigue, blood pooling, intolerance of exercise, headaches, blurry vision, palpitations, tremors and nausea.

After years of testing and waiting, I'm finally closer to getting answers, but unfortunately, diagnosis isn't usually quick or easy when it comes to chronic illnesses.

~

Let's head back to the beginning of my orthostatic symptoms and delve into yet again another lengthy diagnostic process.

From a young age, I would develop bright (almost neon) orange and pink splotches on my legs after showering or standing for long periods—we first assumed unknown allergies were causing these "rashes". My arms and legs frequently went numb, and I became dizzy when I stood up from lying down, or after I got out of bed in the mornings.

I swapped all my products for sensitive skin ones, trialled various shampoos and conditioners, tried antihistamines... but none of this helped. We couldn't figure out what was wrong, so we were forced to carry on and hoped I never had a worse "reaction".

Later, as my Tourette's and FND developed, I began learning about other conditions as well as my own. I researched chronic illnesses, memorised everything I could about my symptoms, and I spoke to many other people with different disabilities too.

After discussing my symptoms with friends who also suffered from dysautonomia, they suggested that I should get tested for POTS. I showed my mum some information about the condition and we both agreed that it could explain nearly *all* of the symptoms I'd had since childhood. We then contacted my GP, who referred me for further investigation.

As you've probably learned throughout this book so far, waiting lists are one of the biggest barriers to getting diagnoses in the UK, so this was yet again something I had to face. Alongside my ongoing FND diagnosis journey, this new referral was over-whelming. I attended so many appointments—none of which were giving any answers. I was eventually seen by a cardiolo-gist, and he performed an echo of my heart.

"An **echocardiogram**, or "echo", is a scan used to look at the heart and nearby blood vessels. It's a type of ultrasound scan, which means a small probe is used to send out high-frequency sound waves that create echoes when they bounce off different parts of the body."
- NHS

I had these scans frequently when I was a baby, because I was born with a small hole in my heart. This caused a heart murmur to develop (I have an extra "da dum" beat in my heart!) and this had to be monitored until I was about two years old.

But, aside from the known murmur, this scan was normal, and we were once again left with clear scans and no answers for my symptoms. My next test was an ECG (electrocardiogram) which is where little wires are placed on different points around your chest to monitor and measure your heart's waves. This is similar to an EEG (which I had during my investigations for Tourette's and FND), but this time to monitor my heart.

"An **electrocardiogram** (ECG or EKG) records the electrical signal from the heart to check for different heart conditions. Electrodes are placed on the chest to record the heart's electrical signals, which cause the heart to beat."
- Mayo Clinic

I want to share a funny story from my ECG appointment because it makes me laugh—and cringe—every time I think about it! The light-hearted glimpses in between stressful moments are important to share, because appointments aren't *always* negative or traumatic. I want to reassure people that it's okay to laugh and have positive experiences, even during tough times.

You are allowed to celebrate the times where you *do* get help and you *are* listened to, even though we mainly speak about complaints of the healthcare system. There are hundreds of thousands of amazing doctors and nurses, and many patients receive life-saving and life-changing treatments every single day. We should celebrate these moments too!

During an ECG a few years ago, a nurse came into my room with wires to be placed on my chest. My first thought was… but, how do they put the wires on under your top?

At this point in time, I had just turned sixteen and was therefore still uncomfortable with my ever-changing teenage body. The thought of taking my top off was horrifying! I thought the nurse was joking until my mum widened her eyes to silently imply, "What are you waiting for? Just do what the nurse says."

Scans or medical tests can definitely feel nerve-wracking if you haven't had them before, but I am here to say it does get a little easier with practice. The more appointments you attend, the more you interact with nurses, and the more tests you have, the easier it gets to normalise it all.

I will *always* go bright red if I have to reveal my body for something like an ECG, but I'm slowly accepting that doctors have seen *much* more embarrassing and revealing things and probably wouldn't remember my face after the appointment.

After making a compromise, I covered myself with tissue paper and continued with the ECG. A nurse attached the wires, and I sat quietly until another doctor came into the room to take the ECG readings. The technician kept looking up at me and I awkwardly smiled whilst my tics chattered away.

During an ECG you have to stay as still as possible to get the most accurate reading, therefore this proves an enormous struggle when you have Tourette's. I tried my absolute hardest to suppress any tics for those few minutes, but this usually results in my tics worsening afterwards. I began swearing and making rude gestures to the doctor, but thankfully he didn't mind. He understood that tics are involuntary and knew the anxiety from the scan was making my tics more active.

After we finished the scan—me still sat holding a piece of tissue paper over my chest—the doctor asked about my hobbies, and whether I'd ever made videos on TikTok. I went a shade of red brighter than you can imagine. I said, "Yes... I actually make awareness videos for my conditions and show people my life with tics" and waited for his response. He then admitted to seeing my Covid test video and said he'd actually watched a lot of my videos. How embarrassing! Talk about awkward moments for somebody to recognise you from the internet, right?

We ended up chatting more—*after* I went back behind the curtain to put my top back on—and my mum was nearly crying with suppressed laughter. My face still shone bright red, but I managed an amusing conversation with the technician in between bursts of tics. We talked about my content, my plans for college, and then I told him about a song I was recording at the time (this song was "She's Mine" for those of you who have listened to my music—it's available on all streaming platforms if you'd like to hear which song I'm talking about!). I ended up playing a recording of my song to the nurses and they all loved it!

This was a *bizarre,* funny, and overall quite positive experience because of the lovely staff members. Although I still get embarrassed when thinking about that appointment, it's a memory that never fails to make me laugh.

≈

After a few more months of tests (including an ambulatory ECG which is the same test, but done over 24 hours where you carry the machine and wires with you) and getting more "clear" test results, the doctors still had no cause for my worsening symptoms.

My episodes gradually became more frequent and significantly interrupted my daily life. I started to faint nearly every single day which only worsened during my health flare-ups. Whilst still waiting for a diagnosis, I spent my days lying on classroom floors, trying not to faint but inevitably failing each time. I'd put my legs up, drink water, and try to breathe calmly, but the faint always came when I stood up again so I felt hopeless!

Eventually, my ECG results came back... only to report no "worrying" episodes except a few jumps in heart rate which were marked as not concerning; we were back to square one. Since I'd already been seen by my local cardiology department, I was referred to a specialist POTS clinic as my doctors believed this was the most likely diagnosis. We once again waited months for a phone call, and then even more months for my first investigation: a tilt table test.


My mum and I took the train to the specialist clinic two and a half hours away. I remember feeling dreadful on the day, both mentally and physically. My symptoms were acting up, and my OCD was so bad that I became increasingly frustrated.

When my body isn't feeling great or I'm flaring up, I often feel even more overstimulated than usual, which leads to increased meltdowns. Textures, sounds and smells overload my brain with information, and everything feels like it's *wrong* and I can't fix it. I feel too many emotions at once, yet I struggle to identify or understand the emotions I'm actually feeling (this is a common autistic experience called alexythmia), I just know I feel really, really crap.

Despite all the struggles, my mum planned the whole journey and we treated it as a girly day trip. We spent some time in a bookshop and had a cup of tea in a cafe near the train station which helped to make the day feel less clinical and overwhelming.

The specialist clinic was like a maze! Hospitals often have lots of floors and if you haven't spent much time in them, it's incredibly easy to get lost in the endless corridors when they all look very similar. There's usually limited daylight in the inner wards and —especially with public holidays or the pandemic—hospitals are often overwhelmingly crowded. This is extremely stressful to cope with, so please don't judge yourself (or anybody else) for feeling overwhelmed or intimidated.

Going to the hospital on your own (or even with other people) can be frightening, and it's often a recipe for meltdowns with all the beeping machines and constant moving, talking, doors closing, pens tapping, different clinical smells and harsh lighting. If you can, try to take deep breaths and ground yourself so you don't get caught in the rush of the environment—staying calm and regulating yourself could make the difference between having a positive or negative experience!

After eventually finding the cardiology department, my mum walked me into the consultation room to help explain my tics and health history, because I'm notoriously terrible at talking to doctors.

This may come as a surprise due to my videos and how articulately I advocate for my conditions online, but during medical appointments I often experience verbal shutdowns. This isn't something I've talked about much on social media but I want to share this in case people reading can relate or learn something new. My mum mostly does the talking for me, and I add in any details that haven't already been mentioned. I also use written lists to help remember what I need to communicate. I sometimes show these lists and notes to people instead of verbalising, especially if I'm struggling to get my words out or feel too overwhelmed to talk.

After settling in and going through my information with the nurse, my mum had to leave the room and we began the test.

A tilt-table test detects any heart rate and blood pressure changes when going from lying to standing. This is usually done by strapping you to a bed (whilst lying down) and using harnesses to keep your torso and legs in place as the bed moves into a vertical position. Doctors put an ECG monitor on your chest and limbs as well as blood pressure cuffs on each hand and foot along with a fingertip heart rate monitor. All of the devices are connected with wires that send all the information to a computer for doctors to look at throughout the test.

When the nurses were preparing me for the test, the pulse oximeter couldn't actually detect my heart rate due how terrible the circulation was in my hands—after sitting for a long time and standing in the cold shortly before, my fingers had turned purple. The nurses put heat packs on my hands to raise my body's temperature and get the blood flowing enough to get a reading.

When we started the test, the bed slowly lifted from a lying position to a standing position with me still strapped to it. My body felt so strange because I couldn't quite touch the floor but was still held upright by the straps—it felt a bit like floating. This strange feeling was soon replaced with anxiety as I had to try and keep as still as possible, and the nurses weren't allowed to talk to me due to the effects it could have on my heart rate. The room wasn't allowed to have any decor or signs because taking in information can make your heart rate spike due to emotional reactions, so I had to stay still and stare at the completely blank wall in front of me.

I'm not going to lie, it was *boring* and felt like the longest hour of my life! And yes, I said hour, because tilt table tests are one *whole* hour of just standing and waiting for your blood to pool whilst being strapped to an upright table in a dark, silent room. How fun! (That is very sarcastic for those of you who need the clarification.)

Only a few minutes into the test, I started to feel severely dizzy and reported this to the staff. I told them every time I felt a new symptom, and these symptoms worsened as time went on. My head felt fuzzy, my eyes blurred, my vision went shaky, my legs started to burn really badly and I struggled to stay awake.

My arms felt painfully numb and tingly, but I wasn't supposed to move them due to it interrupting the readings—this was really difficult with my Tourette's as I couldn't let any tics out. My whole body felt like it was bursting with symptoms, emotions and my tics as I tried to suppress everything.

Suppression isn't healthy for people with Tourette's because holding our tics in and trying to remain still can actually result in worsened tics after the suppression period passes. This usually looks like a tic attack for me, where I will have many tics all at once and can't control my body as it jerks and stretches in many different painful directions.

Not everybody's tilt table test will be like mine, but I personally had an awful experience due to the symptoms I experienced, and the fact I wasn't very well in general at this time. Having to trigger physical symptoms for a test is never pleasant, because you do have to actually *feel* those symptoms. I honestly didn't think I'd last the entire hour, but time slipped away as I dissociated due to the pain and discomfort, and suddenly they were lowering the bed back down, untying me and taking the monitors off.

The rest of that day was more symptomatic than usual, which is normal if you've had a test that exacerbates your symptoms for the purpose of getting medical readings. I recommend always taking a day or two of rest after you have a tilt table test because going back to your daily routine too quickly could result in burnout or feeling even worse. I know it can be hard, but allow yourself to rest and recover. Try to be patient with yourself and your body.

~

After months of waiting for test results (*again*), I received a phone call to summarise my previous scans, blood tests, ECGs and the tilt table test. This phone call came at an unexpected time when neither me and my mum had prepared a list of questions (you can find a list of helpful preparation ideas in the previous *Appointments Advice* chapter) which meant that this phone call wasn't very successful. I struggled to advocate for myself and in less than ten minutes, the doctor said that "no symptoms were reported during the test" and that I was being discharged. What?!

I felt *so* disheartened, and was yet again, back at square one. If you've ever had the *joy* (sarcasm) of undergoing medical investigations, you'll know how disappointing it is to find out you're being discharged without answers.

It's not that we *don't* want clear results—it would be incredible to be symptom-free and healthy—but that we still *experience* horrible episodes without getting the answers we'd hoped for. Receiving a negative or clear test result when you're still experiencing debilitating symptoms can be difficult to hear, because it means you're back at the beginning of finding a reason for feeling so unwell.

Luckily, we managed to request another follow-up appointment with the POTS clinic and a cardiologist was patient and willing to explain everything. He went through my whole case, discussed symptoms, listened to me as I explained my history, and then he told us about something called **Orthostatic Intolerance** (OI). After going through my notes and test results, he concluded that orthostatic intolerance was the name for the pre-syncope symptoms I'd been experiencing since childhood.

> **"Orthostatic Intolerance** is the medical term for symptoms that can occur when people stand up, or try to remain in a standing position for more than a short period of time."
>
> - *Dr Charles Shepherd* (ME Association)

I now know that my body doesn't react well to postural changes due to my heart struggling to pump blood around my body fast enough. When I stand, the blood stays in my feet rather than being pumped up to my brain which causes dizziness, blood pooling in my limbs, blacking out upon standing, fainting, fatigue and more.

Despite not having a definitive diagnosis yet and not yet reaching the end of my own journey, it feels good to finally understand why my body works this way. I can also research any symptoms or management strategies because I know more about what's happening.

Below are some of the symptoms of orthostatic intolerance.

- Light-headedness or dizziness (usually upon standing or after sitting with legs below your heart)
- Blurred vision
- Weakness or muscle fatigue
- Inability to stand for long periods
- Fainting (syncope)

- Confusion
- Nausea
- Muscle tremors
- Difficulty concentrating

OI can happen occasionally in a person's life due to many different causes, or it can be experienced due to a chronic condition. Usually when standing up, a person's blood pressure decreases slightly because blood pools in legs. Certain cells in the body sense this change in blood pressure and adjust the heart rate to pump more blood back up to the heart, thus stabilising blood pressure.

However, in somebody who suffers with OI, this process malfunctions and causes our symptoms. This malfunction can be due to (but not limited to) dehydration, prolonged bed rest, heart problems, thyroid conditions, diabetes, an excessive intake of drugs or conditions such as POTS.

I want to share a few tips from my personal journey which have helped to improve my circulation and decrease my symptoms. There are many other ways to manage dysautonomia, but these are the most common recommendations which I've personally implemented into my own life to help reduce symptoms.

Remember that you should never change your treatments or take medication without seeking proper medical advice from your doctor! Changes and treatments will work differently for different cases, so every person's body will have slightly unique needs.

## ADVICE FOR MANAGING ORTHOSTATIC INTOLERANCE:

**Wearing compression stockings.**

These help to increase blood flow from the feet and legs to the heart and brain. I find these socks to be immensely useful! My symptoms typically reduce when wearing compression socks, so this is a life-saver if I know I will be standing a lot, or sitting with my legs down below my body. You can also get compression leggings which go all the way up to your torso; these may increase the positive effects as more blood is pushed back up to the heart and the brain.

**Getting plenty of fluids.**

I'm terrible at this one (hands up if you're constantly dehydrated, because me too!) but staying hydrated and increasing your water and electrolyte intake does really help with blood flow—thus increasing brain function.

**Avoiding alcohol.**

This helps a lot of conditions including my FND and Tourette's, but I've heard many people with POTS and OI also recommend this.

Alcohol is a poison, meaning when it's ingested, your body has to work even harder than usual to try and rid your body of the toxins. Adding this process to your body's daily "to-do list" uses up vital energy and can lead to worsened functioning (a.k.a one hell of a hangover).

You should do whatever suits your lifestyle, but this could be something to discuss with your doctor to see if it could help reduce your symptoms.

**Increasing salt in your diet.**

Please speak with a medical professional before changing your diet because I am not a doctor and I do not have access to your bloodwork or notes! I can only share what I've personally experienced, however increasing salt is something that most doctors along my journey have suggested.

Increased salt intake can help to increase blood plasma volume (more volume of blood to pump around the body) and—when paired with increased water intake—can aid hydration. I naturally add *lots* of salt to my food, so this wasn't a big change for me—I guess my body knows what it needs!

**Light movement or exercise.**

Moving and stretching throughout the day can keep your blood pumping and can help improve circulation. I stretch every morning after waking up and every night before I go to bed, as this helps me feel less stiff or sore after being stationary throughout the day. Movement is especially important if you're a wheelchair user, you work from home or you spend a lot of time in bed because the less mobile you are, the less your muscles are working, therefore it's more difficult to maintain strength.

It's important to find a careful balance so you keep your body moving and healthy, whilst not worsening symptoms by doing *too* much. Monitor your symptoms and do whatever feels good for your own body. Try to listen to any cues and do what your body is telling you to—whether that's rest, movement, getting fresh air, or a light stretch.

**Getting up slowly.**

This sounds obvious, but if you feel dizzy upon standing and struggle with blacking out or fainting, then standing up more slowly could help you. I always sit upright a few minutes before getting out of bed so that my posture changes as carefully as possible. This can prevent vision from blacking out and reduces the risk of falling. Changes like this can take a while to get used to, but it's a good habit to build to keep yourself safe.

**Tracking your heart rate.**

Heart rate tracking devices can be extremely useful when trying to implement pacing, and learn which activities affect your body the most. For people with POTS who suffer from tachycardia (high heart rate), being alerted when your heart rate goes above a certain beats per minute can help prevent fainting episodes and allows you to treat symptoms earlier.

You can measure heart rate using most smart watches, but using specialised devices such as the *Visible* band can be even more useful for people with chronic illnesses, due to the pacing and symptom tracking features available in their app.

# TWENTY-TWO
# TIC FEST & SEIZURES

As I settled further into college and distanced myself from past negative friendships, I started to see improvements. My focus narrowed in on my social media advocacy and hobbies because I simply couldn't *do* much else on bad health days.

College was incredibly lonely—I didn't go out with friends and I felt increasingly isolated as I focused any limited energy on my studies. But on the flip side, having social media as an outlet did allow me to meet some truly amazing people and I'm incredibly grateful to have had the online community during my hardest times.

Posting content enabled me to make friends, and the internet also introduced me to communities like support groups. Tourette's Action (the UK charity for Tourette's syndrome) hosts events every year where people with TS can stay with other people with TS for a few days. They hold "Tic Fest" events for families, "Adult Tic Fest" for over 18s, and also "Teen Fest" which is a smaller event for teens aged 14-17.

After a few years of not being well enough to attend, I finally worked up the courage to book a place on a Teen Fest event in the Lake District (a national park in the north of England). I was SO nervous in the months running up to the trip, and constantly prayed my health would be good enough to let me go.

Despite my difficult time during college, this retreat in 2022 changed my whole perspective. It was my first time meeting people in real life who'd struggled with severe tics like me, and also my first time being in a room with so many people who all had Tourette's! Everybody had different tics, different stories and different lives, but when we all arrived on the first day it was like we all *understood* each other.

Parents don't stay with you during Teen Fest events, so I said goodbye to my mum and settled in for two nights. I didn't know any other people there so, as a fairly socially-anxious person, it was definitely out of my comfort zone!

After some awkward introductions and a *lot* of tics, we got to know each other and shared some stories about our lives. We realised a lot of us had similar tics and often related to each other's experiences; being able to finally relate to somebody felt incredible. It's extremely valuable to meet people who you can relate to, because as a disabled person we often feel like the odd one out in a crowd, or that we never quite fit in with everybody else. But on this trip... I felt like I belonged.

I instantly clicked with one of the other girls called Erin. She was really funny and made me feel welcomed and comfortable straight away, I knew straight away that we'd be good friends. There was also somebody who had FND too, so we talked lots about our experiences as I'd never met anybody with FND before either!

On the first day of camp, we settled in and played some games (including a very noisy, chaotic game of twister which involved many tics) and then we roasted marshmallows around a fire in a big teepee tent. The staff made us feel included and safe, which was a positive change from feeling like a liability on school trips. Since TA retreats are designed specifically for people with TS, all of the dangers are taken into account and planned for.

Staff offered to roast marshmallows for anybody with dangerous tics or who didn't feel safe around the fire, and they made us feel confident letting all of our tics out judgement-free. I honestly forgot I was ticcing most of the time because everybody was doing the same thing! I didn't register my tics as embarrassing or out of the ordinary, even though they were *more* active than usual due to being triggered by seeing other people ticcing.

The scenery is beautiful in the Lake District. We had the most breathtaking view of the mountains in the distance, and I did some gymnastics moves in front of the sunset while we were playing games outside in the fresh air.

The next morning, we took a mini bus—which was very loud with all of our shouting tics—up into the mountains to do something called ghyll-scrambling. If you've never heard of this before (I hadn't either!) then it basically involves climbing up part of a mountain, but instead of taking the path... you climb up the river. We had to wear huge wellies (waterproof boots) which I found difficult due to my OCD not liking to touch other people's things. It was a mental battle to put on the borrowed boots, but I managed to keep calm, focused on the activity, and actually had a lot of fun!

I recorded this whole trip for my YouTube channel so if you would like to go and watch this in a visual format and see what I'm describing, then you can actually watch along in between reading! We climbed up steep waterfalls, through gushing water, jumped into a deep section of the gorge, and hopped across steep rocks with no ropes—which was pretty terrifying but definitely very exciting.

One thing neurotypical people often don't know, is that seeing people tic or being around somebody with Tourette's can trigger our own tics. This means that our tics become much more active when around other people, presenting a whole new challenge to living with TS.

Due to the constant amount of tics around me, my own tics gradually wore down my energy until my body started to shut down—this is where my other condition, FND comes into play. Functional neurological disorder often worsens during times of extreme stress or tiredness, so it usually kicks in when my tics push me to exhaustion. It's sort of like my body needs a break, and can't continue any longer, therefore my brain shuts off and stops functioning correctly—like a computer short-circuiting.

This shut-down happened at Tourette's camp because my body was so exhausted from all the tics and excitement that my FND symptoms kicked in. Despite the positive and fun moments, my evenings on this trip were spent unconscious due to constant seizures.

On the first night, my seizures weren't too bad except for a few minor episodes (which were a daily occurrence for me at the time), but on the second night, my health took a turn after settling down for the evening.

I remember sitting in the communal space trying to watch a musical on the TV. I chose to sit on the floor because I was feeling "strange" and wanted to be near the ground in case I needed to lie down or I fell.

I don't recall much due to the fuzziness experienced before and after seizures, but the other people said that one moment I was sat up, just silent and not moving (this is an absence seizure which usually happens before I have a bigger seizure), then the next moment I fell and dropped into a full convulsive seizure in front of everybody. In any other place this would be extremely embarrassing for me, but I actually felt safe here due to how understanding and kind everybody was.

The staff were calm and handled any seizures without panicking, which made such a big difference! Making seizures feel less scary and more "normal" actually makes them a lot easier for us to cope with, because we don't have to worry about people's reactions. It also helps to keep us calm which can actually reduce our symptoms at times.

After a few longer seizures and multiple head drop seizures, I began to black out and wasn't regaining consciousness in between seizures any more. One of the other teens walked me back to my room, standing beside me as I brushed my teeth in case I fell.

On the way back to my room, I suddenly fell in the corridor into another convulsive seizure. My friend caught me as I fell, which saved my head from injury thanks to their impressive reflexes!

I only recall the events after this due to a video being taken. I often ask my friends to record my medical episodes because this is useful for my doctors and it's reassuring for me to know exactly what happened while I was unconscious. I'll describe this video to you as it made me feel very safe and loved.

I was lying in the corridor mid-seizure, and somebody put my favourite teddy (I take my panda, Benji, with me on every trip) in my arms so that I could hug him even while unconscious. Looking back, this was so sweet and I appreciated the gesture a lot. People also put pillows around me to prop my head up, and turned the lights off to make it feel more calm. One of the staff members stroked my hair and spoke in a calm, soft voice, which is the perfect way to respond in my opinion.

People's reactions to seizures can make a big difference for us in the moment, and it affects our mentality when waking up from an episode. If we're in a loud, judgemental or panicked environment then we'll probably feel unsettled and unsafe, whereas if we wake up with a soft and reassuring voice, a pillow under our heads and our comfort teddy in our arms then we'll probably be in a much more relaxed state.

Seizure first-aid changes depending on the person and the nature of their seizures. For somebody with epilepsy, a seizure could be a dangerous and life-threatening situation that needs a more urgent response, but for my seizures, I need a calm and relaxed response to help me ease out of the episode and prevent further symptoms.

It's best to ask anybody in your life who may have seizures what they'd prefer you to do, so you can deal with their symptoms in a way that suits them. If you come across a stranger who's having a seizure, then here are some common seizure first-aid tips to hopefully better help the person you're with.

## SEIZURE FIRST-AID:

1. **Check for any dangers**, glass or breakable objects around the person, being careful that your surroundings are safe for both you and the person having the seizure.
2. **Move any objects** away from the person so they can't hurt themselves if they're convulsing.
3. Check the person is **breathing,** and that their airways aren't restricted or obstructed. Please never put your hands, fingers or any object inside their mouth.
4. If the person has never had a seizure before, **call an ambulance**. If they have seizures regularly, follow their given protocol or only call an ambulance if they're injured, struggling to breathe, or if the seizure lasts longer than 5 minutes (this is very important for epileptic seizures). *Before doing this, **check for obvious medical IDs** on their person or via medical bracelets

(iPhones also have a medical ID on their lock screen) and follow the directions given if they're applicable.

5. If you can and it is safe to, move the person into the **recovery position** after the seizure to prevent the person from choking. Turning somebody on their side can help to clear airways if the person is aspirating. It can also be helpful to put a cushion or **jacket under their head** if they're on a hard surface. *Do not do this if the person has suffered a fall or a head injury and please follow the directions of emergency services.

6. Note the **time the seizure** starts and ends if you can. This is helpful for paramedics when treating and documenting the seizure.

7. Stay with the person and **talk calmly** to them until they come out of the seizure. Try not to panic or speak too loudly as this can cause stress for the person seizing—sometimes we are partially awake or can hear during episodes.

8. **Report any symptoms and timings to paramedics** or family members when they arrive, as this can be useful for treating the person's condition. Think: *Did they mention feeling unwell beforehand? Was the seizure sudden? How long did the seizure last? Did they fall or hit their head? Were they acting strangely beforehand?*

In the case that a person having a seizure is a wheelchair user, put on the wheel brakes and leave any seatbelt or harness on. Support the person gently if they begin to tip to one side and cushion their head if possible, but don't try to move them as this could make the episode worse or cause injuries.

Additionally, here are some things you should *never* do if somebody is having a seizure.

1. **Never** put anything in their mouths (including your hand or fingers, this could hurt both you and the person in the seizure).
2. Do **not** give the person any food or drink until they are fully recovered as this could be a choking hazard.
3. Do **not** try to lift the person or get them to sit up prematurely—the safest place for somebody who is seizing is usually the floor (as long as no dangerous objects are nearby) to eliminate the risk of falling.
4. Try **not** to panic. This only escalates the situation and can cause more people to become involved, making it unpleasant and overwhelming once the person wakes up and comes around.

Every situation is unique, but these are general guidelines to help keep you and others safe during seizure episodes. Try to stay calm and collected if you can as this can make the difference between a negative or positive experience for everybody involved.

Now that you know a bit more about how to deal with seizures, let's get back to my experience of finding communities through in-person events.

∼

Even with seizures interrupting parts of the Tourette's Teen Fest weekend, we were all given the same opportunities as anybody else, no matter our limitations or any adaptations needed. Nobody asked questions when we needed to take a break or go for a walk to let our tics out, and nobody batted an eyelid when we shouted something or accidentally hit each other due to our tics—it was accepted as the norm.

This is just one reason why events like this are vital for people with disabilities like Tourette's. It makes us feel less alone. We feel understood, accepted, accommodated, and it's the one place where we never have to hide.

Whether you have Tourette's or any other disability, I truly believe it's so beneficial to find a community of people who are living with a similar condition or difference. I found it to be a life-changing experience, and going to that first Tourette's camp really solidified my confidence in my tics!

# TWENTY-THREE
## FINDING PEACE IN MOVEMENT

Although my physical health improved slightly in 2022, I struggled with my mental health more than ever before. I constantly tried to balance mental well-being with college, online advocacy work and all the other aspects of life, but this is extremely difficult when you're disabled *and* neurodivergent. One thing which helped me—and may come as a surprise to some of you—was movement.

The very thing that FND and chronic fatigue had taken… slowly turned into an outlet for me. On my good days, I started doing yoga to stretch my muscles out in the mornings and give me time to breathe and slow down. The gentle and accessible nature of stretching suited me well, and I found I could still do small stretches, even when parts of my body didn't work. I could adapt yoga flows to include only the body parts I could manage, therefore no matter my physical limitations, it made me feel calm and strong.

I spent more time outdoors as spring turned into summer and the pressures of college morphed into the summer holidays. My dad is an avid hiker, so he took me on lots of sunny walks through the forest which felt so good! Getting fresh air always relaxes me, whether it's hiking up a hill or going to the park in my wheelchair.

I love the sound of birds in the trees, the rustling of leaves, the crunching of branches under my feet, and the sound of wind rushing through the grass. Little moments like these help to calm me down. It can definitely benefit our mental health to spend time in nature. To get away from screens and the rush of cities. To just to *stop* and appreciate the things around you.

When I'm outside, I always look around and focus on the tiniest details I can, noticing *everything* instead of letting it all blend into the background. I find this a great way to calm my brain down after a hectic day, because it grounds me and forces me to focus on the present rather than worrying about the future.

I also find water very relaxing. Studies have proven that seeing water or being beside bodies of water (lakes, rivers, or the ocean) can actually make people feel happier! I didn't believe this at first, but now I've experienced the impact of being in nature for myself, I can definitely understand why it can improve people's well-being.

Life can feel heavy, especially with mental or physical challenges, therefore finding these little snippets of relaxation and happiness does make life feel a little more "worth it". Within the neurodivergent community, a common term used to describe these moments is a "glimmer" which was coined by psychotherapist Deb Dana to explain the complex poly-vagal theory.

> "Glimmers refer to small moments when our biology is in a place of connection or regulation, which cues our nervous system to feel safe or calm."
> - Neurodiversity Education Academy

On the theme of positive moments in life, I'd like to share

some positives from the past few years, because it's definitely time for an uplifting chapter! Here are some highlights and things I achieved despite all the challenges I had to face, both mentally and physically.

For Tourette's awareness month in 2022 (15th May to the 15th June), Tourette's Action set a challenge to raise awareness for Tourette's and fundraise money for the charity. For this challenge, I decided to do one hundred sit-ups every single day.

Although the final video never saw the light of day (sorry, YouTube!) I filmed my sit-ups every day to document my experience and to hold myself accountable. I remember being on holiday at Centre Parcs (forest holiday parks located around Europe) and every night before bed, I'd grab a cushion and complete my one hundred sit-ups just to prove to myself that I could. And I did!

It's strange looking back on this now that my health has progressed and limited my movement more, but I still feel incredibly proud of completing this challenge. Every day, I accomplished a task that not only made me feel good, but had a greater cause like fundraising which could help other people too.

I highly recommend setting small goals or challenges for yourself, even if it's just getting out of bed or stepping outside once a day, because having that goal and mindset can help increase motivation and make you feel capable, even when your mental health isn't great.

This doesn't have to be a physical challenge (many of us can't complete these because of health conditions, and that's okay!) but rather something like drawing, painting one picture every day, writing a poem a day, or another hobby you enjoy. Every year, I complete a writing challenge called NaNoWriMo where you write 50,000 words during the month of November, so this may be an idea for those of you who like writing stories.

Also in May of 2022, I completed a challenge where I ran 100 km in a month to raise money for *Great Ormond Street Children's Hospital* (GOSH for short). GOSH is one of the world's leading children's hospitals (located in London) and specialises in children's healthcare, finding new and better ways to treat childhood illnesses. This hospital sits very closely in my heart because somebody I love was treated there for many years and received life-saving treatment, so I wanted to give back, even if it was just a little.

My GOSH challenge overlapped my Tourette's awareness month challenge, so life was incredibly hectic for those 15 days. I set up a fundraiser and successfully ran (and walked) 120 kilometres in May... which meant that I actually surpassed my initial goal!

Even though the challenge was difficult, I'm proud of myself for staying committed and doing something that means a lot to me. It feels surreal that I completed such a physically demanding challenge, especially now my health is a lot more limiting, but it really shows how much a person's life can change in a few years, or sometimes just a few months.

I would one day *love* to do a challenge like this again, but my health has deteriorated and I unfortunately can't run due to joint pain and other health issues. However, I still keep active with low-impact activities and stretching to keep my body feeling good.

One way I've incorporated movement into my life in the past few years is gymnastics. Fully circling back to my childhood, I plucked up some courage and went to an adult gymnastics class a few years ago. I am so glad I pushed myself out of my comfort zone to do this because it massively improved my mental health!

As a young child, I absolutely loved gymnastics. I stretched every day, did the splits anywhere I could, and I even added gymnastics moves to my cheerleading routines at school. I had posters up in my bedroom, mats spilling out of my wardrobe, and I attended classes for a while. In late primary school, I quit and didn't step foot in a gymnastics gym again until I was seventeen. But wow, I am glad I went back!

If you had a childhood sport that you fell out of love with, then you'll probably relate to the sadness it brings to think of where you could have been if you'd just carried on. *Where would I be if I hadn't quit and had instead trained hard for all these years?* I definitely had this thought a *lot*.

Something I didn't realise until my first adult gymnastics class is that sports don't have to end with childhood. Granted, I don't put on sparkly leotards or go to competitions with other gymnasts anymore (though I secretly wish I could)... but I did find that same sense of community and found that the concentration of learning new skills for fun was even more valuable than medals or trophies would ever be.


During my first class, I was terrified! I had a few different worries: I didn't know anybody, I hadn't been there since I was about ten years old, I had health struggles to think about, I wasn't sure how much I could do or if I could keep up, and finally... I had Tourette's syndrome and I was walking into a room full of strangers.

Luckily—to my surprise—everybody was absolutely lovely! I made friends on the first day who I'm still good friends with now. It felt easy to chat with people and nobody questioned me when I said I might meow, twitch or say a swear word every now and then.

When I first started, the class was incredibly hard. I'm definitely not as fit as when I was a child, so the movements seemed a lot more intimidating. I had to be careful going upside down due to my fainting issues, and I was constantly afraid of hurting myself on the beams or the bars (looking at them now, kids are somewhat fearless!).

I'm proud to say that after a few months of practising, I could do a few skills including a back walkover and a "flic". If you're not familiar with gymnastics, this looks like a backflip where you jump and bend backwards onto your hands, bringing your feet over your head and then pushing off your hands to land back on your feet. It felt like flying and I realised I'd missed this feeling so much!

My coach Adam never failed to make us laugh (or cry, if we're talking about strength conditioning) and always made everybody feel welcome. When I tore my pec muscle during our first session of 2023, he was really calm and supportive when I couldn't come back for months on end. When my shoulder finally healed, I was so glad to be back so I could chat to my group of gymnastics friends again.

I've missed a lot of gymnastics sessions due to my health, and I'll never be able to do sports competitively. Being chronically ill, I have very unpredictable symptoms and need to save energy in order to manage my health and reduce flare-ups. I was forced to stop all sports and workout classes last year as my health progressed, and this brought a lot of unexpected grief. It felt like losing a part of me, and I wasn't sure how to continue now that my body physically couldn't do so many of the things I loved.

But… I learned that my chronic illness won't stop me from doing things I love—those activities may just look different for me! I will ever stop doing the things I love when I *am* able to do them. I try to move my body whenever I physically can, and I try to fully allow myself to rest when my body can't keep up. Even when I have painful symptoms or my chronic fatigue is particularly debilitating, I still try to do some form of adapted movement both for my mental health and to reduce physical soreness. Adaptations can make most things accessible if it's done in the right way for you!

Movement has definitely helped me through the past few years, and for the first time since being bullied, I can confidently say I *like* being active! I've always loved netball, cheerleading, dancing, gymnastics, yoga, roller skating, hiking, swimming and running. I loved to do all of these things when I was healthy and well enough to do them.

Moving makes me feel good—it makes me feel like I'm in control of my body even when many of my days are filled with episodes, uncontrollable tics, seizures or feeling too fatigued to get out of bed. It reminds me of who I am behind the health struggles and diagnoses I have, and that is incredibly valuable.

After listing my past physical achievements, I want to highlight the inevitable grief that many disabled and chronically ill people go through. The grief of looking at your past self and wishing you could do as much as you used to. Wishing things could be different, thinking "what if" and "if only" and feeling cheated out of a healthy life.

I often feel heartbroken when I see past photos or videos of me running, jumping, dancing, flipping and doing very physically demanding things. I yearn for my old body, one which can allow me to do sports and keep up with the people around me. But I also recognise that this is a normal process to go through.

After writing this chapter, I do wish I could still achieve physical challenges. But the reality is that I can't right now, and that's okay too. My body has changed, my illnesses have become more demanding, and I'm still recovering from the many years of stress and burnout my body was put through.

I can't run, walk around shops, go to gymnastics, do workouts, or hike up hills at the time of writing this, and I haven't been able to for quite a while now. Even as an advocate myself, I still question how my life can look *so* drastically different from how it did two years ago. I question *why* this happened to me, *why* I don't have energy, *why* there's no cure, and so on. There are so many unanswered questions that most disabled people have likely thought of, but it's important not to let these depict how we experience the world right now.

Yes, I wish I could do the things my younger, healthier body could do, but I'm also grateful for all the incredible experiences I've had recently. I can still go out when I'm using my wheelchair, and my powered attachment enables me to go fast and replicate the feeling of wind on your face during a run. I can attend concerts, festivals and events due to accessible venues and disability accommodations. I can laugh, see friends, post online, watch sunsets, and enjoy so many things even when my freedom of movement has been severely reduced and taken from me.

Honestly, this isn't the reality I thought I'd have as an adult… but it's the card I was dealt and it's the one I have to work with whether I like it or not. So, I'm going to do everything I can to enjoy the things I *do* have!

It's important to remember that you are *you*, no matter what health struggles you're facing. There are always ways to keep up your creative, or sporty, or clever side, however that may look to you. Disabled or chronically ill people often can't do things the same way as others (or the same way as our past or younger selves) but it doesn't mean we can't achieve amazing things and enjoy activities.

We are capable. We are creative. We are sporty. Some of us love to dance, whether that's on our feet or in a wheelchair. Some of us love to bake. To crochet. To visit and explore different places. Some of us—like me—love writing and reading books!

We can love anything anybody else can love; being different doesn't change that. Being disabled just means that it's more difficult to access, manage, process, and facilitate activities, and that our methods may look slightly different.


We should, as a society, try to include more disabled representation and inclusion in our acknowledgements of accomplishments. And, I don't mean giving us a prize just for being in a wheelchair and seeming inspirational (this can be incredibly patronising), but actually acknowledging and celebrating that disabled people are strong, creative and successful both *despite* and *with* our differences.

I urge you to read books by disabled authors or listen to music from queer and neurodivergent musicians. Go to an inclusive event, or correct somebody when they use ableist language. Acknowledge that we are people, we are humans and we deserve chances, opportunities, and respect just as much as anybody else.

# TWENTY-FOUR
## A-LEVELS

For those of you who aren't from the UK, college is a two-year period of our education system (between ages 16-18) where we complete A-Level exams. Usually, students pick three A-Levels, but some people may take four, opt for one larger subject as a whole course, or choose an apprenticeship instead.

I chose to study English Literature and Language, Art and Design, and Music Technology—I chose my three biggest hobbies as my main subjects, which was definitely a positive change from the nine subjects in secondary school.

Throughout the first year of college (as detailed in my earlier chapter *Starting College*), I had an incredibly difficult time with my health. I mostly focused on my coursework and my music (both in my Music Tech class and personal projects).

Music has always been a big part of my life, but in college it became even more important to me. I learned how to professionally record the songs I'd written, and I released two of these on streaming platforms for people to listen to. I actually recorded my first (and most popular) song just before college, so that one was entirely self-taught!

As part of my college music class, we learned how to perform and set up for a live performance, which led to me forming a band. I met some other music students and we practised each week after college to prepare for the "Live Night" where students played a concert on the college stage.

Before my band's first performance, I'd never played or sung in front of a live audience, so I remember feeling nervous jitters all over my body—this was made even worse by the added risk of my seizures.

I created a care plan with my music teacher to prepare for any health risks and ensure we had a plan in case anything went wrong during the concert. I highly recommend doing this for events (such as music performances) if you suffer from seizures or health issues. It's always important to be prepared for any circumstances, just in case.

On the day of the concert, I felt increasingly unwell in the run-up to the show because the added stress of performing made my symptoms worse. Luckily, I survived the performance without any mishaps and I successfully performed alongside my band! I played lead electric guitar and even did a solo which received a huge round of applause and shouts from the audience—it felt amazing!

This is definitely a big highlight of an otherwise difficult time at college—and throughout the first year of college, I performed another two times and even sang lead vocals in one of the concerts. I will always be proud of myself for getting up on the stage and doing what I love.

Focusing on my hobbies made life feel a lot less miserable amidst dealing with physical symptoms. If you suffer with a mental or chronic illness (this also applies to everybody), I highly recommend finding activities you enjoy, because having distractions, no matter how big or small, can help divert your attention to something positive rather than focusing entirely on your health. In my case, this massively improved my mentality.

At the end of first year, revision season began. Unlike all the other students, I couldn't spend my time revising in the library or doing homework like most other students. My time outside lessons was occupied with rest and dealing with the aftermath of exhausting episodes. I quickly fell behind and missed more and more deadlines. My grades started to drop quite rapidly.

I'd always been a straight-A student before this, so it was a shock to my people-pleaser brain when I started getting Cs on tests, and even failing to sit some exams. I felt like a failure, and as more and more work was given to us, my progress only slipped further down.

Due to other factors, the stress of health, and my college work, my mental health hit a crisis point in 2022. I pulled away from everybody and stopped doing the things I enjoyed. As a way of coping, I focused entirely on just getting through the days one at a time, and only *just* managed to keep myself afloat.

~

This is when I started sharing videos of my worsening FND and dysautonomia episodes, documenting the faints and seizures which interrupted most of my classes.

I was in my English classroom one day (sitting next to my best friend of many years, Megan) when my vision suddenly cut out. It was like time stopped and then suddenly, I was back in the room and feeling fuzzy. When I refocused my eyes and came around, everybody had moved. I realised entire minutes had passed.

This is what it can feel like to have an absence seizure, and I still experience these on a daily basis. Sometimes they can last a while and may come in clusters, causing a lot of disruption in my memory and concentration, whereas on other days I may only have one or two brief episodes. If the absence seizure is short and nobody around me notices, I sometimes don't even realise it's happened! This is why I record any episodes where I'm alone or outside of the house, as I can watch the videos back and see what happened. It's useful to know the timings of seizures and whether I had any other symptoms during the time I was unaware or unconscious.

In college, I started having more, and more, and *more* of these episodes until I could hardly remember what I was being taught. As summer approached, I hadn't retained much information from classes, meaning I had to re-teach myself all the topics. I looked through PowerPoints outside of class and spent every spare moment revising in an attempt to keep up. It felt like constantly chasing my tail and never catching up with it. This is when we decided to request a meeting with my college.

It wasn't my first meeting (and it certainly wasn't my last) but here we put in place the new changes which enabled me to stay in college. My mum and I brought up the scary possibility of dropping out, while the staff discussed moving back a year, repeating college, dropping one or two of my subjects, moving to an online school instead of in-person… we discussed all of the possibilities.

I truly thought there was no chance of me finishing college and getting my grades as planned, at least not on-time. I felt defeated, and like a lot of chronically ill people whose academic potential is halted due to health or mental health, I felt like I'd failed even though it wasn't my fault.

In the end, my college reduced my timetable and implemented online lessons for whenever my health was flaring up. I didn't attend any assemblies, I had no social life, I spent lunchtimes at home, I didn't go to RE classes or registration, and I had to leave all of my clubs, including choir.

Losing my hobbies was particularly tricky to process as I'd been in choirs every single year since primary school. It was like I had to give up a part of me purely to keep my head afloat, and this was difficult to adjust to. It felt so unfair!

With chronic illness, it can often seem like we're going backwards in order to move forwards, but I can assure you that this feeling is normal, it's necessary, and it is *okay*.

Post-diagnostic regression is something I also experienced after my autism diagnosis due to all the accommodations I realised I needed. I couldn't spend hours shopping any more, I couldn't sit in a classroom due to the sensory overwhelm, and I struggled to communicate more than ever before. I felt "more autistic" than prior to my diagnosis. But this isn't because these traits *suddenly* appeared or worsened, it's because I hid and ignored my needs for so long that I simply couldn't mask them any longer.

With a disability (for example, my Tourette's and FND) our needs can increase or decrease at any time. Symptoms can chop and change in frequency and severity, which leads to different capabilities depending on how we are feeling.

Not being able to do something that you used to doesn't make you any less of a person, and you shouldn't feel guilty for taking a step back or reducing your workload.

～

After reducing my timetable to only my basic lessons, I had additional time to rest, allowing me space to do college work and also sleep off any exhaustion. Hurray! Exam season passed, and although my mental health was still declining, I successfully made it through my first year of college.

On the last day, my mental health hit a breaking point and I finally reached out for help. There's a lot I haven't shared online and much more I probably won't ever share publicly (it's important to keep boundaries, especially when trying to keep safe online) but this was a *very* difficult and low time for me.

I spent most of that summer trying to keep myself busy and distracted from my constantly whirring brain. It may be evident in my content from that year, but there were a lot of moments where I lost myself. I lost my fashion sense, my hobbies, my social life, and I felt the least "me" than ever before. I didn't even know who that person was anymore.

Mental health can impact your life tremendously, and it can define the difference between living and barely surviving. Your perspective and outlook on the world change due to chemical imbalances, environments, or other factors. This can make you feel like you're completely alone, like the world is too big of a challenge to face.

Mental illness can impact anybody, anywhere, at any time. It doesn't matter if you're talented, successful, or if you've never struggled before in the past; mental illness can affect any person regardless of their background. This is why it's so important to speak up and check in on the people around you, even if they seem "okay" at the time.

That summer, for the first time in five years, I started therapy. I accepted help at a point of crisis and after only a few weeks, I had an appointment with a new therapist. I'm beyond grateful for finally having a positive therapy experience after years of feeling like I couldn't trust anybody.

When I was thirteen, I had a counsellor who I didn't bond with at all. She broke my trust, and I learned to shut people out for years. But this time, I instantly clicked with my therapist and as I slowly began to trust her more and more, I told her everything.

I can't express in words how opening up truly did change my life, but it did! Therapy was *not* a quick fix and I definitely have more things to work on, but speaking up and accepting help was the start of my recovery journey and it led me to a much better place.

If you don't find your first therapist useful, then I'd highly recommend trying to find another therapist if you have access to it. Different therapy and talking styles work for different people, so not everyone will have a positive experience with the same therapist. Some people may have enjoyed working with my counsellor from secondary school, but personally, it only pushed me further back.

It's okay to try things and find out they don't work for you, but don't let this rule out everything else. It's okay to learn from experiences which didn't suit you, because you can take note of what did and didn't work, and keep trying new options.

The rest of my 2022 is a black hole in time. A lot of mentally ill or chronically ill people may relate to this analogy, but my days slowly blended into one big clump of struggling and lots and lots of tears.

Breaking down my mental walls (which I'd had up for so many years of my life) was incredible progress in many ways, but it also unleashed emotions I wasn't quite prepared for. It seemed like I struggled even *more* after opening up, but in reality, my struggles were just outwardly shown rather than hidden.

When I struggled with feeling overwhelmed, I vocalised it and asked for support. I talked through my emotions instead of shutting myself in my room and pretending everything was okay. I spoke up if I was overwhelmed, and this helped to reduce sensory overload. To others, it looked like I could tolerate less and less, but in reality, I was just speaking up for things I'd always struggled with internally.

Breaking down that mental wall opened up an immense amount of internal work I had to do, and this was immediately overwhelming. I sometimes still get the urge to slam that wall back up and rebuild the "safety net" of pretending I was fine. When I wanted to feel capable, my natural response was to hide and mask my feelings.

But I learned—through many breakdowns and nights spent in tears—that there is only so much time you can spend pretending that everything is okay. There are only so many years you can spend following the influence of others until you become so burned out you can't function anymore. There are only so many times you can go through friendship breakups until you question whether you're capable of keeping friends at all. And there are only so many times you can tell yourself you're fine until you realise that you were never *truly* fine at all.


I've realised through many conversations with my therapist, best friends, family, my journals, or through online conversations with people like me... that I am not a failure for struggling or for admitting I'm not as "fine" as I used to be.

It's okay to feel like you've regressed when you begin listening to your mind and body and actually begin managing your needs. You are **not** alone!

# TWENTY-FIVE
## GOODBYE EDUCATION

My second year of college flew by, as I was busy catching up on classwork, sleeping, recovering and just bobbing along however I could.

Sometimes chapters of our life aren't exciting or productive, but instead are necessary breaks or focus periods we need in order to progress and recover. I made lots of progress with managing my health needs during this time because I finally focused more on myself and prioritised health over any social expectations.

In my second year of college, I completed Music Technology exams which involved mixing live music for the college concert. I sound engineered for a few of the bands and helped set up the stage too. I also managed to get a live sound role for my college's production of 'Little Shop Of Horrors' which was an incredible experience!

I was the only person in my year helping with the audio mixing, so I had exclusive access to the box—which is a little room at the back of the stage hall. Inside there were huge mixing desks with many dials, sliders and all the controls for the speakers and microphones. It looks intimidating at first, but I quickly applied all the knowledge from my classes and successfully helped our technician run the show. This was one of the brightest and coolest memories from college, and it's something I'll always look back on.

Even with my health struggles and the pressures of staying afloat in classes, small glimmers were always present. These moments are the important parts of life; they're what keeps us motivated, wanting to carry on and push through hard times.

After my music exams finished, I spent most of my time revising for my upcoming English exams. Due to health flare-ups and mental health struggles, I'd missed a *lot* of work… but I made it through to spring. I finished my Art and Design course after creating an entire children's book for my final project. I wrote a story and illustrated digital art for each page, which I then made into a full physical storybook!

I remember having two tic attacks during my art exams which were caused by being in a quiet room with everybody else. We had to be supervised during exams (and the art supplies were in the art rooms), therefore I had to sit in the classroom instead of in learning support like usual. This arrangement came as a surprise to me, and I worried a lot about how I'd cope with the quiet environment with my tics being loud or distracting. I used earplugs to distract myself from other people so I didn't have to worry about how loud my tics were, but sometimes this isn't effective if my tics are particularly active.

When I'm struggling with depression or feeling low, my tics lessen or become quieter as I lose my excited and cheery nature. Contrastingly, when I'm happy and excitable, my tics are loud and become more active with intense emotions. During my A-Levels, my tics were mostly 'meows' and other small sounds or words because my low mental health reduced the severity of my tics—this allowed me to concentrate much easier than I could for my GCSEs.

However, in one of my art exams I began to feel incredibly anxious in the silence. I could hear everybody's breath, the sound of their pencils, the clock ticking. The whole room filled with tiny noises which pounded inside my head. I gradually became more aware of my loudening vocal tics and panicking when people began to notice.

My echolalia tics (repeating other people's words or sounds) started to copy my teacher, who had a sniffle and was coughing. Every time he coughed or sniffed his nose, my tics would repeat the sound in the exact same way. This happened again and again, and again, until everybody on my table was trying not to laugh. Even though it's light-hearted looking back on that tic, it felt so embarrassing and frustrating at the time. I just wanted to concentrate on my work and be quiet! I couldn't control my tics, which meant I felt completely out of control.

As I said before, intense emotions usually result in tics worsening, so this stressful exam understandably triggered my Tourette's. I left the room and made my way to the toilets— taking one of my permitted rest breaks—but when I got into the bathroom, my tics only got worse. I couldn't breathe due to the coughing tics, which made me feel even *more* panicked. My tics were hitting my chest and shouting, my arms jerking out in all different directions and hitting the walls. I slipped into a full-blown tic attack.

I find it useful to document episodes so I can look back on them and notice any triggers or unusual tics, and it also helps people better understand my conditions when I share videos of my experiences. Sometimes it's hard to watch videos of tics (or can even trigger our own tics, which can make it difficult for people with Tourette's to watch other tic content), but tic attacks are a reality I've always tried to include in my content where possible. I want to show the genuine experiences of Tourette's, including both the good and the bad. I try to make my content accessible for everybody while still depicting the harder sides.

After this episode, I went home early due to the exhaustion and had to finish my exam another time (this was pre-arranged in my exam preparations, so I highly suggest planning for situations like this in your school care plan!) when I'd recovered enough to go back into college.

We later requested permission for me to use headphones in my art exams, even though this isn't usually permitted because of the risk of cheating. Playing background music helped to calm my tics and anxiety, so the following exam sessions were much easier.


My final subject was English Literature and Language, my most "academic" of the three. I had multiple written exams which (with my additional 25% extra time) lasted over two hours each. These required a lot more preparation and concentration than my other subject exams, but after spending weeks focusing all my energy on English revision, I completed my exams in a small room in the learning support department.

I'm thankful to say, they went surprisingly well! I felt a massive weight lift off my shoulders when I left each exam. I'd been building up to this stressful period for two whole years, and it was finally coming to an end... I couldn't have been more relieved!

On my very last day of college, I remember packing up my bag after finishing my final exam and walking out into the college's courtyard. The sun was beaming down—first signs of the summer holidays peeking through—and I practically danced across the car park as I made my way to my mum's car.

I couldn't believe college was over! All of the days spent with my head in revision books and exam papers was finally over, and I immediately felt lighter. I climbed into my mum's car and gave her the biggest smile, before driving home and asking myself "what do I do now?" as I thought of the months ahead of me.

# TWENTY-SIX
## BRANCHING OUT

I'd directed all of my energy towards college for two years... so when I finally finished, it actually left me feeling quite lost. I didn't have a job like other people my age, I didn't have any hobbies or clubs due to focusing on exams, and I'd lost touch with most of my friends when I was too unwell.

I was still recovering from severe health flare-ups and a mental health crisis, so I *definitely* wasn't ready to jet off travelling on a gap year or head to university like other people in my year. Honestly, I remember thinking *'what the hell do I do with my life?'* after arriving home from my final exam.

I spent many weeks resting and not doing much at all—this was very necessary and I highly recommend allocating time to do this—after the exam period, and it quickly reflected in my health. My seizures slowly lessened from multiple daily to one every few days, and my mental health improved as I focused on getting myself better and doing what I enjoy. I didn't have to spend my energy worrying about grades any more!

In hindsight, I strongly believe that leaving college was the key to making my life more enjoyable and liveable. Leaving education was the catalyst for finding myself, finding out how my brain works, and learning how to work *with* it rather than battling against it.

If you're currently questioning your decision to take a gap year or you're considering taking a year out to focus on your health or mental health, I recommend to *DO IT!* Take all the time you need to focus on yourself and make sure you know how to work *alongside* your conditions before diving head-first into work or university.

Despite finishing education and feeling less stressed, my mental health was the worst it's ever been. My college life is a time I will never forget, and not because it was good or memorable, but because it's the lowest I've ever felt. Much of that second year is blurred out of my head. We all have good and bad days and low and happy times, but those of you with a mental illness will relate to having severe rock-bottom moments in life. This was probably mine.

After distancing myself from people during health flare-ups, I didn't have an in-person social life beyond my family. This was made even more difficult due to my undiagnosed autistic struggles, which made it nearly *impossible* for me to find and keep friends.

I didn't know who I was, who I was meant to be, where I wanted to go in life, whether I'd ever get a job, whether my hobbies were "worth" my energy, and so on. I hope some of you reading this can feel comforted in knowing you're not alone—though I wish nobody had to relate to these difficult and isolating feelings. I hope for all of you to one day feel joyful and settled again. Just know that it *is* possible to find your path. You can (and with time, will) find your purpose, your people, your way of working, and most of all, you can find things that bring you joy again.

It's sometimes hard to admit quite how much you've struggled, especially in a world full of expectations to achieve, grow, and be successful, but that's exactly why I want to share my experiences in this book. It's hard for me to write abut my lowest and most vulnerable times—knowing people will read this all over the world—but I know some of you will relate to this and feel a little less lonely. This thought alone makes everything I do 100% worth it.

∾

I received my A-Level results later that summer (somehow achieving an A* in English, A in Art, and Distinction* in Music Tech!!!) and was freed from all ties to education. After weeks of resting and recuperating, I finally felt ready to branch out and begin my new journey beyond education, beginning with… my eighteenth birthday!

I became an adult on the 20th of July—just after finishing my exams—and I still don't feel like a "real" adult, even now. My birthday was a quiet celebration with a few of my closest friends. I felt an immense pressure to conform to the usual drinking, partying, clubbing and big social stereotype of eighteenth birthdays, but that just isn't *me* at all.

Since learning that I'm autistic and making an effort to accommodate my brain, I've stopped forcing myself into activities I don't like purely fit in with everybody else. This was my first step in doing things I *actually* enjoy rather than the things I'm expected to. I've found that keeping a close, small circle of friends works best for me, and this has saved me the stress of maintaining friendship groups and living in that constant cycle of drama-filled friendships. I'm more than happy with just a few people to spend my time with—my best friends are the most incredible humans in the world. I love you guys.

I'm still on a journey of discovering what works for me and what I like to do, but the further I grow into my unmasked self, the more I branch out and re-discover how I can enjoy life. And yes, that does include socialising!

Shortly after my eighteenth birthday, I took a trip down to Oxford, which was my first time travelling since becoming chronically ill and losing independence. My mum drove me to the train station, and I met my friends from the Tourette's community, Jess and Anouk. We explored the city, spent time together, filmed videos and enjoyed the lovely weather.

Only a week or two later, I took the train again, but this time to London (the busiest city in the UK). This next trip taught me a *lot* about my needs whilst travelling, so—after flaring up for months due to the chaos and upheaval of this particular trip—I want to share the adaptations I use to make travelling with health conditions a little bit easier.

## TRAVELLING WITH DISABILITIES

1. If you have physical disabilities or mobility struggles, **take your mobility aids**! For this London trip (my first time visiting the city in years) I didn't take my wheelchair or my crutches, which I now know was a *big* mistake. I assumed I wouldn't need them because I could walk unaided at the time of leaving to catch the train. The issue with this is, that travelling usually *triggers* and worsens chronic illness symptoms— therefore, by the time I'd travelled, done a day in London, attended an event and socialised for hours on end, my symptoms badly flared up… right in the middle of the event. On recent trips, I've prepared much more sensibly by taking my mobility aids, whether that's my wheelchair, crutches, or simply planning places to sit and rest during the trip.

2. Book **travel assistance** at the airport or train station. I'd never used any form of travel assistance before recent years—but let me tell you, it is an absolute lifesaver! The UK has travel assistance for trains called

'Passenger Assist' which can be booked in advance on the train's website, or via the app. I book assistance every time I travel, and it's made travelling so much easier. You can request a wheelchair space, a transport buggy, companion seats, and staff can help find your platform, navigate crowds, find your seat, and carry luggage for you.

3. Take your **comfort items**. Whether it's safe foods or a pillowcase to reduce sensory issues, taking comfort items can make travelling go a lot smoother. I personally take lots of comfort items with me even for one-night trips, because I know I'll have that peace of mind when I'm away from home. My usual packing list includes: a pillowcase, my own cutlery, a flannel, comfort clothes like a hoodie, my panda teddy, and lots of other day-to-day items like noise-cancelling headphones, earplugs, fidget toys, and my sunflower lanyard.

4. If possible, **bring somebody with you**! Whether it's a parent, carer, friend or just somebody you can trust to support you, having another person to help out can make the difference between safety and danger. Even if your conditions don't cause immediate danger (for example, experiencing seizures where you could fall and hit your head), it can still be unsafe to travel on your own if you're disabled in other ways. Having somebody to help navigate or communicate for you can reduce misunderstandings with tics, prevent autistic meltdowns, save energy if you suffer from chronic fatigue, or can just make your journey less stressful.

5. For many modes of transport, you can purchase **disabled discount cards** which could entitle you to cheaper fares for both you and a carer. In the UK, you can purchase a Disabled Railcard for discounted train

travel, which is especially helpful when you need to bring more people or luggage due to your conditions.

~

My London trip the summer after my A-Levels was my first time attending an event as an "influencer" for my online advocacy work. How exciting! I attended a Disability Pride Month event hosted by TikTok and spent the evening in a room filled with lots of other disabled and neurodivergent content creators and advocates.

This event marks a huge mindset switch I had with unmasking and accepting my disability. After many difficult years—and isolating myself from people—I'd definitely lost touch with my identity when it came to disability. I'd stopped posting videos of my seizures, avoided taking photos in my wheelchair, and I was neglecting my needs by pushing myself way too far, way too often. But… this trip broke me free from this mindset completely.

I met the most wonderful humans who all embraced their disabilities with such pride and confidence that I felt completely at home. I felt like I'd found *my people* for the first time in my life, and I spent days feeling emotional and thinking about this moment. It was like my world suddenly clicked into place and I re-discovered my passion for advocacy that I'd lost during my mental health decline.

It's okay to doubt yourself or to have ups and downs with your confidence, we all do! Even I (a disability advocate) have moments where I feel like I'm not valid or that I "should" be doing more than my body currently lets me. There are moments where I wish my life was different, where I feel like giving up, and moments where I don't want to see myself as disabled.

But, I've realised there is so much talent and goodness within all of us, no matter what we've been through or what conditions, labels or differences we have. If we search for it, we can find that acceptance we need within ourselves. We can find a community. We can find people who make us feel our best, and who provide us with adaptations, accommodations and acceptance. And slowly, we can also find this feeling within us, accepting ourselves for whoever we may be.

This event marked progress for me in terms of socialising, but it definitely took its toll on my body. By the end of the event, my legs couldn't hold me up and I struggled to stand at all. My FND kicked in along with the familiar feeling of seizure warning signs, shaky legs and tremors. I instantly knew I'd pushed myself too far.

After leaving the event with my friend Seren, we had to walk to the tube station in order to get home... but this was much easier said than done. This may just be my biggest disability trip fail yet! Seren is blind, therefore I was in charge of navigating the centre of the biggest city in the country (which I wasn't familiar with), in the pitch-black night.

If you know anything about anxiety, social anxiety or autism, then you will probably recognise the dread that comes with navigating new places. This situation gave me that feeling times ten! There were road closures, meaning our phone GPS sent us down dark alleys with no street lights, and we ended up going to the wrong place not once, but twice. It was a disaster. The whole time, my legs were crumbling underneath me so Seren held me up with her arm and we limped along as heavy rain poured from the sky.

If you take anything from that story, please let it be this: plan, plan, *plan*! Planning is especially important if you have to manage a chronic illness alongside all the other challenges of travelling and navigating new places. Before any trips, make sure you have steps in place for if your health worsens, and take any aids or medications with you that you may need in an emergency. It's *always* better to be prepared than to be caught off-guard and find yourself in a pickle.


As you can probably guess, this busy summer of birthdays, trips and events caused a flare-up and left me feeling unwell for months afterwards. I used my wheelchair most of the time and I couldn't get out of bed on a lot of days. This is the reality of travelling (or doing any taxing activities) with a chronic illness: it's unpredictable, sometimes scary, and can have really brutal consequences afterwards.

But, despite this, disabled people *can* travel! It's important for people to remember that we can do things that others can, and we deserve to have those opportunities. We can explore, enjoy social events, play adaptive sports, and take part in *most* activities non-disabled people can. Modern adaptations are incredible and enable us to branch out further than ever before, giving us some of the freedom that non-disabled people naturally have.

Accessibility isn't perfect (it's far from it) but there are still many ways disabled people can be supported and given alternative options when our conditions or surroundings are limiting. You deserve to take part and enjoy things, even if it looks different for you or needs to be adapted into a more accessible version.

# TWENTY-SEVEN
## NEURO-DISCOVERY

I could honestly write an entire book about this next journey (there is so much I could talk about), but I'm going to share a brief insight into a part of my life I've only recently understood and accepted: being diagnosed as autistic.

Following the months where I lost my identity and even started to regress in social skills, I finally began to open up again when I started the process of an autism diagnosis.

I started researching into autism (also known as ASD or ASC) in 2021, shortly after finishing secondary school. Before talking to some other autistic women online, I had no idea about how differently autism can present in women and adults, especially those who are high-masking. For months, I researched day and night until I slowly discovered people who I could relate to through online videos. I finally felt seen… and I suspected I was like them too.

The thought of reaching out and applying for a diagnosis was daunting at first. Autism doesn't have a very positive "reputation" in the general public, and it's often misunderstood and under-diagnosed. I'd heard stories of autistic people being denied access to places or denied adequate healthcare, and I'd grown up with school kids who had patronising and negative attitudes towards the word 'autism'.

At some point in history, neurotypical humans decided that being autistic was a bad thing, and the word slowly became an insult. Growing up, the word 'autistic' was used as a synonym for "weird" or "abnormal" which only pushed autistic people further from the bubble of social acceptance. This is not okay.

Being autistic is not a negative thing, though autism does come with a lot of frustration and struggles for many of us. We shouldn't be shamed purely because our brain processes information in a different way, or because society is set up in a way that is catered to brains.

We don't need to be fixed, and we don't need to change in order to fit in or to appear neurotypical. We need support and accommodations. We need acceptance. We need sensory-friendly spaces and better education systems. We can thrive and live much more happily if we're supported and helped through any struggles, rather than being cast aside and forced to conform to a box we don't fit in.

After speaking to numerous autism advocates and other autistic women, I built up the courage to accept that maybe I *was* autistic, and maybe that wasn't a *bad* thing! Autistic friends taught me that their diagnoses helped them to understand themselves and allowed them to grow rather than shrinking or hiding.

Along with reaching out to people online, I continued going to therapy throughout 2022 and 2023, which helped immensely in my unmasking journey. As I learned more and more about my needs, I slowly found my place in both the disabled *and* neurodivergent communities. I found hope that an autism diagnosis could be a lightbulb moment for me too.

*So* many questions came up during this process. *Maybe I wasn't weird or abnormal? Maybe my differences and "flaws" were actually autistic traits? Maybe I wasn't a bad friend, and actually just communicated differently? Maybe there are other people like me out there? Maybe, I wasn't actually alone?*

Again and again I made lists (endless lists should have been an obvious sign from the start!) about autistic traits which matched me on every diagnostic website I could find. It took two years of heavily researching and talking to other people for me to accept that I **was** in fact, actually autistic.

Self-diagnosis is a topic that many people feel uncomfortable talking about. It's often seen as "taboo" because of the hate people receive when they share their experiences online, but it truly shouldn't be this way for autistic people. In the UK, our NHS waiting lists for an ASD diagnosis are incredibly long, leaving over 140,000 people waiting for an autism assessment in England as of December 2022.

> "86% of people (121,000) waiting for an autism assessment in England have been waiting longer than 13 weeks."
> - National Autistic Society

Getting a medical diagnosis is not accessible for many people, and this leaves them without explanation or validation of their struggles. So many autistic children and adults are put onto waiting lists where it can take up to a few *years* to receive an assessment, leaving them without support for far too long.

I was put on a waiting list for an ASD assessment in 2022, and I didn't hear anything back until around October 2023. When finally receiving a letter, I was so excited to hear some news after

ZARA BETH

waiting for what felt like *forever*. But when I opened and read the letter, my heart sank.

It stated that all adult services in my area were disbanded, and that there would be no service available for up to five years. You read that correctly, *five years*! I was so disheartened and cried to my mum, knowing that my already slim chance of having a positive diagnostic experience was slipping away. I read the letter further, and saw that I couldn't apply for an assessment via any other geographical area because I'd already applied locally, meaning I had my hands tied. They couldn't offer services where I lived, but because I'd already enquired, I couldn't apply to a different area either.

This experience left me feeling so disheartened as I'd already waited months just to hear back about getting an assessment. I'd researched so much, analysed my childhood during question-naires with my therapist, and talked to my mum about my traits so much that I was *confident* I was autistic. The signs were there, and the traits explained my previous struggles perfectly. It explained my brain!

I knew in my heart that I was autistic, and that this realisa-tion untangled so much of my life that I hadn't understood before... however I couldn't get a diagnosis to "prove" it.

This is why autism self-diagnosis (when thoroughly researched) is valid. People who have spent years outlining their own traits, struggling to explain them, researching for months on end until they feel they are confident enough to finally say "I think I'm autistic", deserve validation and recognition!

Self diagnosis doesn't happen after watching one TikTok video and deciding that you "now have autism" like many people believe, it's a lengthy process of many months spent agonising over every single detail of our lives until the knowl-edge is solidified that our brains do in fact, work differently from neurotypical ones.

I didn't feel comfortable posting about being autistic until I got an official diagnosis, mostly because of how large my platform is. I'd been scrutinised for years when posting about having Tourette's syndrome (despite being officially diagnosed), so I was terrified of people telling me that I was wrong or that I was faking. This shouldn't have to be a worry for autistic people. We know our brains better than anybody else, because we live with them! Every single day we experience *our* lives through *our* minds and eyes, so surely that gives us the ability to know exactly how we perceive the world?

Trust your gut, trust your intuition, and trust your research— because adequate healthcare is not readily available to every-body. We should encourage and help people to find answers so that they can understand and accommodate their traits and needs to make their daily lives easier, even without an official piece of paper.

If you're going through this process right now and doubting yourself or you're worried about judgement from others, please know that you are not alone. And that you are VALID!

# TWENTY-EIGHT
## MAKING IT OFFICIAL

So, getting a formal autism diagnosis… how did it happen?

In early 2022, I was referred for an autism (ASD) assessment through the NHS, however as I explained in the last chapter, this didn't end successfully. My local services were closed, and I'd already waited nearly a year at that point. I quickly grew tired of waiting, feeling like I had to hide my true self purely due to a lack of healthcare access. I didn't feel validated enough to talk about my own experiences until I had a piece of paper telling me that I was in fact, *correct*. As many of you will know, this is an incredibly frustrating situation to be in.

Around this time, I attended more neurodiverse events and connected with more autistic people which further solidified my suspicions for myself. I began to finally say—out loud—that I was autistic!

This seemed like a *huge* deal at the time. I was so scared to label myself as autistic because I feared people would ask me for "proof" of diagnosis. But thankfully, my friends, family and the autistic community all accepted me as I was! They listened to the things I struggled with, tried to adapt and offer accommodations where needed, and people accepted my "new" discovery surprisingly well.

I chose not to disclose this online until much later, and I'm glad I decided to wait. I needed time to get used to the discovery myself! It takes many days, weeks, and months of going back over every struggle in your life, unpacking traumas, re-thinking every social conflict or panic attack you've ever had and questioning "could that have been autism?" to finally begin your acceptance journey.

It's important to note that an autism diagnosis and acceptance journey looks very different for everybody, and this is only *my* experience. Lots of people are diagnosed as children, or perhaps not diagnosed until their late adult life, so please never judge anybody's experience based on one other autistic person's perspective. As many people say, if you've met one autistic person, then you've only met *one* autistic person.

After I concluded that I definitely felt 'at home' in the autistic community and that I was finally on the right path, I started to research into alternative diagnostic routes like private healthcare. This is obviously not accessible to everybody, and I'm extremely grateful I had the privilege of financial savings to spend on getting a diagnosis I desperately needed.

I researched different organisations, different price points, spoke to other autistic people who'd paid for private consultations, and I finally settled on a company recommended to me by a fellow autistic content creator. I contacted them, asked about their services (they were lovely and explained everything I needed to know, very autistic friendly!) and even had a call with them to discuss how their assessments worked. After feeling confident that they would treat me well, I decided to go for it.

I have created many videos about my whole journey including all of the details about my own assessment, so if you'd like to know more about the company I went with and how online assessments work, feel free to head to my social media using the QR code at the back of this book!

Spending hundreds or thousands of pounds on a diagnosis may seem unnecessary to some people (especially if you're reading this as a neurotypical person) but to me, getting a diagnosis was a lifeline.

As I've said many times in previous chapters, finding out I was autistic changed everything for me. My perspective changed, my confidence increased, I finally gained genuine friends, and I no longer felt like I was alone. It gave me a path to follow that I *actually* understood, therefore getting an official diagnosis allowed my brain to finally begin healing. It allowed me to move on.

I feel it's important to note here that although finding out I was autistic was positive in many ways, it did also bring up a *lot* of emotions. It was difficult to finally discover and accept the reason I'd struggled my entire life. I felt a deep sadness for my younger self who never felt like she fitted in, and had no idea why. I felt cheated out of a "better" childhood where I could have understood my needs and accommodated for them. I felt completely and utterly lost, as I dove head-first into a new world of neurodiversity—I had no idea how to feel or how to even *begin* sorting through the mess inside my head.

∽

My private autism assessment was fairly speedy in comparison to usual NHS healthcare in the UK. There weren't any mega-long waiting lists, so the process only lasted a few months from start to finish.

I spent the weeks before my assessment collecting evidence (doctors' notes, lists, writing down all my traits and struggles) and filling out all of the pre-assessment questionnaires. I had to answer *many* multiple-choice questions which revealed things I'd never even considered could be autistic traits. I learned a surprising amount about myself through this process and uncovered both childhood and teen struggles I hadn't linked to being autistic before.

When the day of my assessment came, I was *so* nervous! My tics became active with the emotions running through my body, but my psychologist was very understanding. After introducing the call, she revealed that she was actually qualified in *both* autism and FND—she knew what FND was! It was the first time I felt validated for both of these conditions, so this appointment was memorable in many ways.

In medical appointments, FND patients are frequently misunderstood and invalidated due to misconceptions and lack of knowledge about the condition. In addition to the planned autism assessment, my psychologist also explained about how FND can link with autism, and how the two diagnoses interact with each other. Hearing validating facts which explained my previous struggles and diagnoses felt like she'd explained entire life in just one call. This helped to change my perspective about my health because most of my struggles with FND, anxiety, OCD, depression and eating struggles… all linked and interacted with being autistic.

> Please note that autism is a separate diagnosis from both FND and Tourette's, and my autism does not explain or link to my Tourette's. These diagnoses *are* common to have alongside each other due to being co-morbid, but they are still separate conditions where people can have one condition without having the other.

FND is not caused by autism, but the two can definitely interact and influence each other. For example, if I'm particularly dysregulated and suffering from autistic burnout, then my FND symptoms may increase because my brain is under significant stress. Similarly, now I'm aware of being autistic (therefore managing my triggers and sensory needs more adequately), I've found that I can better manage my FND too.

I am generally a lot happier and mentally, I'm doing the best I've been since childhood. Read that sentence again… my mental health is the *best* it's been since being a *child*! I'm confident in this being due to finally understanding the way my brain works.

As you will have guessed, my autism assessment did indeed diagnose me as being autistic! We discussed my whole life, including friendships, relationships, struggles, achievements, school life, mental health, coping mechanisms, rituals, sensory difficulties, panic attacks, meltdowns and everything else we could think of. After we logged off, my mum and I actually burst into tears at the sheer emotional load of what we'd just discussed and found out.

Both the assessment call and my confirmed diagnosis were positive in many ways, but it was also incredibly overwhelming. Being autistic, I tend to feel overwhelmed a lot faster than other people, therefore the impact of discussing such huge, emotional, and life-changing topics was a lot to digest. I scheduled a few weeks away from socialising and content creation just to form a plan and file away all these new feelings and findings.

I highly recommend taking a post-assessment break if you have the ability to. Even if you think you're prepared and already know you're autistic like I did, the assessment process and emotional load of receiving a diagnosis can still hit you like a ton of bricks. I was convinced I'd be able to carry on as normal after my assessment (I thought I would suddenly accept myself and finally unmask fully!) but unfortunately, the truth is that it's *not* quick or easy.

Getting a diagnosis is a huge step in accepting yourself and living your life in a way that suits you, but it's only *one* step of the way. There's a whole staircase of further steps in any journey of accepting yourself, telling other people, learning to adapt to your needs, learning to *recognise* your needs, and so on.

I'm still in the process of understanding myself, and I'm constantly learning new ways of accommodating my needs (and discovering new needs or struggles) even now. Most people keep learning even *years* after their diagnosis, so don't rush yourself into anything. Take time—as much as you need—and slowly let yourself come out of the shell you've been in for so long, but be patient with yourself when the outside world feels a little more difficult or unnatural at first. If you've been conditioned to hiding behind a mask (or in your shell) for a long time, then suddenly breaking out of that is going to feel awkward and difficult, but with time you can adjust to the changes, and so can the people around you.

Post-diagnosis, my life changed a lot in a short space of time. Outwardly, not many things changed (except my fashion sense coming back), however there have been countless internal shifts happening.

I've become almost *lighter* because I can finally explain the way I feel. I have a reason why I struggle and interpret things differently from others. I've started to accept that my energy levels and social battery are different from other people my age, and that is okay. I've learned that traditional "fun" social events don't always suit me and that I don't need to participate in ones I don't particularly fancy.

I've started to accept myself for whoever I am instead of using other people as a guide; I no longer mould and shape myself into the "perfect" person for others. I've found daily accommodations for my sensory needs, like wearing sunglasses inside shops (even when it feels silly) and wearing noise-cancelling headphones any time I'm outside the house.

I've finally let people in and found friends who I "click" with even when I'm not trying to adapt myself to their interests or preferences—they like me for just being me! And finally, I've opened up to my family, friends, therapists, and even started sharing my identity and self-acceptance journey online.

Opening up and being honest used to terrify me, because I didn't know who I was or how I was supposed to behave without copying other people. I had no idea what colours I truly liked or what fashion sense looked flattering without my friends *telling* me. I didn't have confidence in myself—mentally or physically—and it felt like every social attempt ended in a big burnout filled with misunderstandings, arguments and failures.

But since learning why I feel and work this way, I now have perspective that I've never had before. When I'm struggling or feeling "outside the bubble" in situations, I can zoom out and look at the situation as a whole, while taking into account my autistic traits. This helps me logically and rationally figure out social cues or identify the reasons I'm struggling whilst showing myself patience wherever needed.

Acceptance doesn't change overnight, and I still get overwhelmed A LOT. I frequently misinterpret or misunderstand both myself and other people, but now that I know and understand *why* this happens, I'm able to pick it apart and put a plan in place for the future. I finally feel like I can stand on my own two feet and just enjoy living without constantly worrying about whether or not I fit in, because I've learned that sometimes standing out is even better.

# TWENTY-NINE
# FINDING YOUR PEOPLE

It can sometimes feel impossible to fit in when you're neurodivergent or disabled. Our bodies don't function well enough to keep up with the fast-paced rush of everyday life, meaning we often miss out on opportunities and social occasions. We're often seen as "difficult" or "boring" for not going out late at night because we know we'll flare up afterwards, or for not enjoying parties because they're too stressful for us. But these struggles or preferences aren't flaws, and they are *not* our fault—they shouldn't automatically be seen as a bad thing!

When you finally find people who accept you (and I promise, they're out there!) you *will* be accommodated for and accepted without having to push yourself beyond your own limits. Genuine friends won't expect you to push yourself past your breaking point in order to keep up with *their* expectations of a busy lifestyle.

True friends ask you how you're doing and they actually listen when you say you need to slow down or take a rain check. They give you space when you're overwhelmed or too unwell to socialise without draining every ounce of energy you have left. They schedule time for you and offer to find times which work for both of your lifestyles, keeping in mind that some hours or days may be difficult with a chronic illness or disability. Kind and considerate people definitely do exist, and there are so many of them out there waiting to be found... just like you.

I personally know what it's like to feel you can't socialise. To feel that friendships always fail and that maybe I'm just "bad" at being with people, but trust me when I tell you that there are *always* people out there who do fit with your lifestyle and needs.

Sometimes we may have to look for friends online (or in a different town or city) because neurodivergent people can be harder to find than your average classmate or co-worker. But don't let this scare you away from finding your people, because they do exist! And when you find them, you won't have to worry about being accepted or accommodated for—it will just be a given.

One of my most prominent examples of finding community was at a neurodivergent event celebrating the launch of Ellie Middleton's book 'UNMASKED' (which is an absolutely incredible resource, by the way) a few years ago. Ellie is a friend I met through the online neurodivergent community who helped me when searching for my own autism diagnosis. A huge benefit of having friends who have been through similar experiences to your own is that they can give you their experience and advice to provide perspective on your own life.

This event was incredibly eye-opening for me as I met lots of autistic and neurodivergent people in-person for the first time. It allowed me to meet the community I'd found online and proved that similar people *are* indeed out there.

We talked for hours and hours about our lives, our struggles, our diagnoses (and lack-of, in my case) and we reassured and validated each other despite having only met a few hours before. Initially, I was taken aback by how enjoyable this event was, because I usually crash-and-burn within an hour of socialising in a "normal" neurotypical setting. However, I found that social-ising with people who communicate in the same way that I do (autistic and otherwise neurodivergent people) actually allows my energy to last a *lot* longer—and I didn't spend the entire evening overthinking my interactions like usual.

People responded to everything I'd shared with "me too" and "I feel the exact same" or "you are completely valid" which felt incredibly welcoming. Multiple autistic women in the room said they'd had the same thoughts and similar experiences, which just shows that we are *never* alone!

Another example of finding community has been the Tourette's events I've been to over the years. TA events are designed for people with Tourette's and they bring a positively overwhelming feeling of being able to "fit in" simply by being around people who understand and accept without judgement.

This feeling of unconditional acceptance is why community events are so valuable for disabled and neurodivergent people (and for everybody!). Community is where we find love, support and friendship—therefore I highly recommend reaching out to people like you (however that may look) and finding people you can talk to.

There is a QR code at the back of this book which links to my social media, website, useful resources, and my Discord commu-nity—which includes forums for many different topics I've covered in this book. There are thousands of people who interact with each other, finding people with similar conditions, talking about hobbies and interests, and asking questions to people with similar experiences.

We have a welcoming and helpful community and I've defi-nitely learned a lot from you guys! I connect with new people in the community every single day—it's truly amazing that the internet gives us a space to do so.

Another community I've found a place in the past few years has been the queer community. I am a proud part of the LGBTQ+ community, which a realisation I finally realised and embraced during my time at college.

Although this isn't a widely known statistic, neurodivergent people are more likely (than the general population) to be gender non-conforming or to identify as queer (this is a generalised term many of us use to cover *all* labels under the LGBTQ+ umbrella). It is estimated that 42–69% of autistic individuals identify as same-sex attracted or as a sexual minority, showing that there is a much higher prevalence than the estimated 3.3% of the UK population who identified as lesbian, gay or bisexual as of 2022.

Terms used for queer people change frequently in society, so please note that 'queer' is a label currently accepted and used by many members of the LGBTQ+ community (like myself) who feel this represents their own experiences better than other labels such as 'gay', 'bisexual', 'pansexual', or 'lesbian'. I personally prefer to use a more generalised term, as I don't feel comfortable choosing one label.

Sexuality (and gender) can be fluid! There is no *right* way to label yourself; whether it's sexuality or gender identity, you should never feel pressured to figure out how you feel or to search for a "perfect" label to explain your own experiences.

For those of you who may not be familiar with it, *gender* is a fluid term which represents socially constructed roles, behaviours, expressions and identities of girls, women, boys, men, and gender diverse people. Gender is different to your *biological sex*, which is assigned at birth as either female or male based on your genetic anatomy.

Much like accepting any diagnosis or life change, accepting your sexuality or gender identity can be a difficult and lengthy process that takes different amounts of time for everybody. It took me *years* of denial to finally accept that being queer was even an option! Everybody's experience with sexuality is different, and some people don't feel attracted to other people at all (this is also known as 'aromantic' or 'asexual') so there is no pressure to figure out your identity or fully understand yourself until (and if) you feel ready to.

In all honestly, I'm still not sure where I sit in terms of labels, despite many years of knowing I was "somewhat gay" after realising I liked women in secondary school. However, I have learned that it is **okay** not to know where you lie. It's okay not to feel comfortable with one particular label and to instead just "go with the flow" and use whatever feels comfortable at that time.

I've personally found that the best way to embrace your sexuality and to enjoy *living* as you are, is to simply just live. I used to put an immense amount of pressure on myself to figure out exactly how I felt in every moment, how I felt about other people, how I should act, who I felt attracted to, and so on. But over the last few years, I've slowly learned that I don't need to explain myself or have everything figured out.

I've grown so much confidence in the process of realising and connecting with my queer identity, and I know many of you reading this may be on this journey too. If you're also part of the LGBTQ+ community, then hello! Thank you for picking up my book, and I hope you feel seen by this segment. I wanted to include a small part of my own story just to highlight that although I mainly advocate for disability representation, I am also a proud member of the LGBTQ+ community.

My online community is a safe space for **all** minorities to find and connect with similar people, because finding people who understood me genuinely changed my life, and I aspire to bring that same validation and comfort to as many people as possible.

Along with my online disability advocacy content, I have also worked with a charity called *The Proud Trust*, an LGBTQ+ youth charity who deliver youth work, one-to-one support, online Live Chat services, and they also manage The Proud Place (Manchester's LGBT+ Centre). This charity is an incredible resource which helps to provide support to young people every single day, and I'd definitely recommend reaching out to similar charities near you to find support, or even ask about ways you can volunteer or get involved.

There are countless challenges we face as disabled people, as queer people, as neurodivergent people, and as a person from any other minority—so it's even more important that we share voices from these communities and help share their stories to the further community.

～

I've done a lot of self-searching this past couple of years. Along with my autism diagnosis and finally opening up in therapy, I truly feel like I'm on the right path—which feels crazy to say after so many years of struggle!

I've grown closer than ever with my family and I've finally found friends who truly understand and accept me. Truthfully, I lost countless friends and had to cut *many* people out of my life in order to get to the place I am now. It took a *lot* of rejection, sadness, fear and some incredibly lonely months to finally start finding the "right" people for me. But when looking back... the journey was *so* worth it.

In the process of distancing myself from unhelpful people and listening to what I truly wanted and needed, I discovered that I didn't *need* other people in order to find out who I was inside. I didn't *need* a friendship group in order to be happy. I didn't *need* to fit in with any group of people, aesthetic, job role, or identity. I needed to figure out what truly made *me* happy.

Even if it seems impossible or scary right now, I'm here to tell you that you don't need to conform to a group or change your-self to fit in with them. You don't need to reference others around you to decide who you are or who you "should" be. You can like whatever you like and be whoever you are, unconditionally.

I've realised that I prefer a 'quiet life' surrounded by slow-paced activities and enjoying the present tense rather than always trying to 'succeed' or 'outdo' expectations. I've found that a couple of genuine friends is all I need, and that traditional cliques or groups don't suit me! I've found that I'm particularly susceptible to mental health struggles, so it's even more important to keep on top of self-care, and to closely monitor my autistic needs to prevent slipping into burnout.

But most importantly, I've found that there *is* hope beyond the endless struggle of feeling like I'll never find my place or find out who I am.

We don't need to have it all figured out! We don't need to know exactly who we are, which aesthetic we fit into, what defines our fashion sense, what sexuality we identify with, which foods we like and so on. It's okay to not know which job you'd like when you're older, or to change your mind once you do get there.

There is a constant pressure to know exactly what you want and who you are, but the truth is that nobody can truly, fully understand or know this. I have definitely fallen victim to the perfectionist, straight-A-student persona in the past, and it led me to feeling extremely inadequate and confused about what I truly wanted. On paper, I was successful and the perfect student, but inside I was crumbling under the pressure. As I've moved into adulthood, I've found this pressure lingers in the new form of finding a career.

Truthfully, I don't know where I will be in a year, or in five years, or ten. I don't know if this will be my job forever, I don't know if I'll move towns or suddenly get the urge to do a degree, or travel, or decide that I don't want to leave home at all... and that's okay. The lesson I've learned from "finding myself" over the past few years has been that I don't *need* to find myself. I can simply just *be*.

Another important lesson I've learned is that although happiness is important to search for on your own (and within yourself), it's also vital to have people around you. I wouldn't be anywhere near the place I am now if it wasn't for my support system around me. I have my online friends and content creator friends, neurodivergent people from all over the world, the tourette's and chronic illness communities, and my entire audience on social media. In-person I have my family, my best friends, my therapists, physiotherapists, doctors (the ones who've given me answers), and also the comfort of my pets.

All of the supporters in my life have cheered me on through countless struggles and journeys over the past decade, and they've helped me guide myself to where I am now.

It can feel scary to let people in and allow them to see your true self—especially if you've been hurt in the past—but when the right people come, it's vital to build those bonds and allow people to help you when you need it. You are not a failure for accepting help from those around you, and it does not lessen the validity of your achievements!

You deserve to thrive and to enjoy everything life has to offer, and I hope with all of my heart that those of you reading this who feel lost right now, can do just that.

# THIRTY
# THE FUTURE

Phew! We've nearly made it to the end. This book has been a roller-coaster of emotions, and it's been both daunting and invigorating to write. I've laid personal things out in writing that I never thought I'd ever tell anybody. I've shared both the hardest and the best moments of my life so far. But most importantly, I've shared my story.

I wanted to give my perspective, experiences and insight so that somebody (hopefully many of you!) reading this can relate to what I've said and feel comforted, so I hope this book has done just that. I want to let you know that those of us who are disabled or chronically ill are also incredibly capable, and that we deserve acceptance, understanding and respect. We deserve to be heard, we deserve to be seen, and many of us deserve better than what we've experienced in the past.

This final chapter is about the future, because that's something I'm feeling excited about for the first time in a very long while.

During all my health struggles, I felt intimidated and quite depressed by the thought of the future. The lengthy span of years seemed never-ending, and not in a good way! I didn't know how to make life seem worthwhile. I wasn't sure what job to do, whether I'd get good enough grades, or whether I'd find friends who actually liked and understood me. Everything about the future is so uncertain, and that terrified me.

However... over the years this has slowly changed, and although the future will *always* be somewhat daunting, I'm feeling excited to see what's to come in the upcoming months and years.

With all the time I've spent reflecting and healing, I finally feel validated in my past experiences. I've finally accepted parts of myself I used to hide, and I'm discovering what *I* like. I'm finally falling back in love with living and I laugh, and dance, and smile again.

Now that I have explanations for why my brain is the way that it is, I also have a better understanding of why certain things happened or why I felt the way I did—and this allows me to better prepare myself for future struggles or situations.

Of course, we can't understand or explain everything, and this is an important fact to acknowledge too. Change is inevitable, whether we like it or not (to all the autistic people reading this, I hate change too) but sometimes it *is* actually for the better.

Transition periods are especially hard when you're neurodivergent, but we can begin to accept the change if we try to remember that it's a temporary period. Transitions come and go, and although the outcomes may permanently alter lives or perspectives, we *will* eventually settle into new routines and situations. It's hard in the moment, and sometimes feels completely unbearable, but in the end we can (and will) always find ways to cope and adjust to our new "normal".

I still have progress to make both mentally and physically, and I will always struggle with my conditions and with being autistic, however, I don't feel weighed down or restricted by this any more. My body and mindset are constantly evolving, therefore I'm working on making my mind strong enough to embrace all these changes and challenges rather than fighting them.

If you fill your life with all the good things and truly acknowledge these little joys, then I believe life can be enjoyable no matter your conditions or differences. It may not look how you anticipated, but there *are* always things to enjoy, even on the darkest of days.


This final and quite positive chapter may seem contradictory to the title of this book, "*Enemy* For a Brain" because it suggests my brain is working *against* me… but let me explain.

My brain was once, in fact, my worst enemy. During my lowest times, I couldn't fathom the possibility of working *alongside* my struggles and finding a comfortable in-between, but it has become easier with time. It does become easier.

I don't know everything. Alas, I'm only human! And I'm still young too. I have so much to learn and hopefully a heck of a lot more to see. But two things I do have… are hope and perspective. And I believe that with these two things (and of course a million *other* things), you can learn to accept whatever is thrown your way and choose to live your life in whichever ways you *can* in order to make the most of it.


My brain did indeed feel like my enemy for a lot of years, however I've since learned that these challenges don't define my capabilities, and my conditions don't define my brain. Yes, I wish my brain didn't misfire signals and stop entire limbs from working whenever stress comes my way… but I've also learned copious lessons from what I've been through. It's been a valuable learning curve and I'm genuinely grateful for all the things I have gained from battling my struggles over the years—whether that's knowledge, talents, patience, adaptability, resilience, community, passion or simply just experiences.

My brain is no longer my enemy. When you start living *with* whatever battles you have, and truly adapting and accepting the reality of them, you're no longer fighting yourself.

I will always be forced to battle Tourette's and FND, chronic illness, painful tics, fatigue, judgement, overwhelm, and burnout. I will probably have **many** more ups, downs, flare-ups, and definitely some meltdowns. But I now know I can and *will* get through them, and I will come out of the other side understanding my brain just that little bit better.

## MY FUTURE (A SERIES OF FAQS)

1. **Will I ever be able to drive?** This is a question I recently discussed with my doctors and neurology team, and it's one none of us can confirm. Right now, I can't drive due to the risk of my seizures, and I've come to terms with that. I'm staying positive by thinking about all the money I will save if I don't need driving lessons, a car, insurance, petrol… plus I get free lifts from friends! There is always a bright side.

2. **Am I going to university?** Currently as of writing this, I'm still in my "extended gap year" (soon to be three years) which was initially intended for recovering from college and prioritising my health after a horrific few years. My first year out revealed so much more than I ever imagined it would—I uncovered the innermost parts of myself and discovered what I truly liked, thought and wanted without the influence of others around me. I explored my fashion sense, fought fears, challenged my anxiety, took content creation as

my full-time job, met new people, and saw new places. After another year out, I finally found a life with balance and I'm working on truly being happy. I know I couldn't have achieved this progress if I were still in education, burnt out and struggling like in my teen years. After reflecting and finding myself on a new path of content creation, advocacy, and writing, I don't think I will ever go to university! I'm not aiming for a job which requires a specific degree, so I plan to avoid student debt and pursue my online career where I can be creative.

3. **What is my job?** I currently define myself as a content creator, writer (hello!), and disability advocate. These things are my biggest interests, and in recent years have become my full-time job. I'm lucky to say that my job is my passion, and it's one which accommodates my brain, my health, and my life as it is now. I'm very thankful to do this for a living, and I hope I can raise awareness and showcase my creativity through photos, videos and projects like this book for many years to come.

4. **How can I be independent with my health struggles?** This is a challenge I'm facing as I delve deeper into adulthood, and it's one I'm not sure I'll ever master. My options are limited due to having chronic health symptoms, but I will navigate each new phase of life as and when it comes. Currently, I rely heavily on my family and friends to support me through daily life: driving me to places, carrying me when I can't walk, staying with me so that I'm not alone, checking in every day, helping me through burnout, advocating for me in hospital appointments when I can't communicate, and so much more. When you're disabled, it can feel impossible to move out, branch out, travel and do all these seemingly "necessary"

things people strive for as a young adult, but I know that opportunities will come when I'm ready for them, so I'm not worried about forcing myself to do everything just yet. Despite this, I am slowly finding accessible and safe ways I can travel, and this gives me a sense of freedom and independence I never thought I'd have. I will likely never be able to live alone, but I'm okay with this, and I know I can be independent in many more ways than simply "doing life" alone.

5. **Will I have these conditions forever?** Tourette's is a lifelong condition, therefore a lifelong diagnosis. It's commonly hereditary (partly genetic) and tics often wax and wane (comes in waves of severity) throughout life. I will always have Tourette's, but my tics may be more or less noticeable at different points throughout the future. FND can also be a chronic condition, however it is unknown what the future will hold for individuals with it—some people fully recover from symptoms, and others live in wheelchairs for the rest of their lives. I am hopeful that my FND symptoms will stay well-enough-managed to live happily provided I'm looking after myself, using mobility aids, and accommodating my needs properly. Being autistic is not a condition you "develop" or something can needs to be cured. Being autistic is who you *are*, it's just one of the many neurotypes. So no, my autism is not "going to go away" or "get better" and I don't need it to disappear! My traits can be frustrating to manage and can be debilitating at times, but with adaptations (and better understanding of neurodivergent needs within society) I hope to be less limited by my struggles and learn to live independently and confidently like many other autistic adults do today.

# ACKNOWLEDGMENTS

First of all, thank you for reading! I'm incredibly proud to have written an entire book. It's unbelievable to think of people reading this all around the world! It's been a *very* long journey of writing this (and years of actually experiencing the things I've written about) so this book is a massive achievement and a stepping stone into a new chapter of my life.

I want to say a massive thank you to all the people I've mentioned in previous chapters and everybody I've met through online and in-person communities who have helped me get to where I am today.

Thank you to my mum, my best friend and co-pilot in daily life —I would not be here without you (literally, lol). Thank you for not only putting up with my chaos over the years, but supporting and loving me through it all. Thank you to my Dad and Kay for sitting through many book-planning sessions, and the rest of my family for being in my life and bringing joy.

Thank you to Stan for being my best friend and partner in life —for always listening, encouraging, laughing, crying, and experiencing all life has to offer with me. You've taught me to love who I am and constantly support me through every up and down. I truly wouldn't be where I am today if I didn't have you by my side.

Thank you to Rosie for getting me through secondary school, for being my rock through hard times and for seeing me when no one else could. To Kylie for laughing with me through college. To Hajrah for constantly pushing me out of my comfort zone and for being my biggest hype-woman.

Thank you to Robin, Daniel, Lucy, Lauren, Jet, and all of my best friends who make me laugh and cry (sometimes at the same time). Thank you for constantly reminding me that it's okay to be myself—you show me the good in this world.

To Evie, Seren, Neve, and all the lovely ticcy humans who have been my sounding board for all things neurology since this all started. To all of my autistic friends who helped me accept my own diagnosis. You have all have taught me many valuable things about how my brain works, and I'm incredibly grateful to have had your support in my journey. Thank you to Ruby, Grace, Zach, Evie and all the team at Tourette's Action for hosting incredible events and leading me to make lifelong friends.

And of course, to my cat Jesse and my dog Lottie for many cuddles and walks when I've needed that unspoken support from a furry friend.

There are too many people in my life to mention by name, but please know that if you've been in my life that I appreciate you, *so much*. You have been invaluable in my journey, and I wish you the absolute best in your own journeys and life's adventures!

And finally, to anybody who has made it this far in the book so far, **THANK YOU**!!! *You* are the reason this community is so positive, so welcoming and engaging. We *are* the community, and together we can help neurodivergent, disabled, queer, disadvantaged and all minorities of people feel heard and seen.

This book contains just one of many voices representing diversity, and it's incredibly important to branch out and support as many different people as we can. You can do this by learning more about disabilities or ableism, de-stigmatising stereotypes, supporting or donating to charities who supply and aid disadvantaged people, and by interacting with posts, reading books, watching videos and supporting the work of autistic, disabled, chronically ill, queer and POC communities.

Keep supporting and checking in on the people around you and take care of yourself too. Do the things you love, chase the dreams that will make you happy, and most of all, *always* strive to be yourself and to love whoever you may be.

I wish you all a lovely day and I hope you go into the rest of your week with a little bit more positivity after finishing this book. You deserve it.

# HELPLINES

Below are some helplines for both the UK and global resources regarding mental health, so that if any of you are struggling with anything I've mentioned, or if you're feeling anxious, suicidal or alone, you have a place to reach out if nowhere else feels safe. You can also find links to charities who support victims of bullying in the UK, USA, Canada, and globally.

**Samaritans (UK)**

To talk about anything that is upsetting you, you can contact Samaritans 24 hours a day, 365 days a year. You can call 116 123 (free from any phone).

**SANEline (UK)**

If you're experiencing a mental health problem or supporting someone else, you can call SANEline on 0300 304 7000 (4.30pm–10.30pm every day).

**CALM (UK)**

You can call CALM on 0800 58 58 58 (5pm–12am every day) or if you prefer not to speak on the phone, you can try the CALM web chat service.

**Mental Health America (USA)**
Call or text *988* or chat 988lifeline.org. You can also reach Crisis Text Line by texting **MHA** to 741741.

**Global Helplines Directory**
To find helplines in your country, visit https://www.helpguide.org/find-help.htm.

**National Bullying Helpline & Website (UK)**
Call 0300 323 0169 or 0845 225 5787 (9am-5pm Monday-Friday) or visit https://www.nationalbullyinghelpline.co.uk/

**Childline (UK)**
Visit https://www.childline.org.uk/

**NSPCC (UK)**
Call 0808 800 5000 (10am–8pm Monday to Friday)

**Bullying Crisis Text Line (USA)**
Text 'HOME' to 741741

**Kids Help Phone (Canada)** - Text 'CONNECT' to 686868

**Crisis Website (Global Information)** - https://www.crisistextline.org/topics/bullying/

# GLOSSARY

**Medical abbreviations & definitions:**

- **A&E** - Accident and Emergency Department (UK)
- **EDS** - Ehlers Danlos Syndrome
- **FND** - Functional Neurological Disorder
- **GP** - General Practictioner (Primary Healthcare Doctor)
- **ME/CFS** - Myalgic Encephalomyelitis/Chronic Fatigue Syndrome
- **NEAD** - Non-Epileptic Attack Disorder
- **NES** - Non-Epileptic Seizures
- **OI** - Orthostatic Intolerance
- **PNES** - Psychogenic Non-Epileptic Seizures
- **POTS** - Postural Orthostatic Tachycardia Syndrome
- **TS** - Tourette's Syndrome

- **Absence Seizure** - Brief, sudden lapses of consciousness which may look like staring blankly into space.
- **Coprolalia** - A type of vocal tic which causes a person to say involuntary inappropriate words or phrases.

- **Dystonia** - A movement disorder causing muscles to contract.
- **Tonic Clonic Seizure** - A type of seizure characterized by loss of consciousness and full-body convulsions.

**Neurodiversity Abbreviations**:

- **ASD/ASC** - Autism Spectrum Disorder / Autism Spectrum Condition
- **ADHD** - Attention Deficit Hyperactivity Disorder
- **ND** - Neurodivergent
- **OCD** - Obsessive Compulsive Disorder

**Other terms used**:

- **EHCP** - Education, Health and Care Plan
- **PE** - Physical Education
- **RE** - Religious Education
- **TA** - Tourette's Action

# ABOUT THE AUTHOR

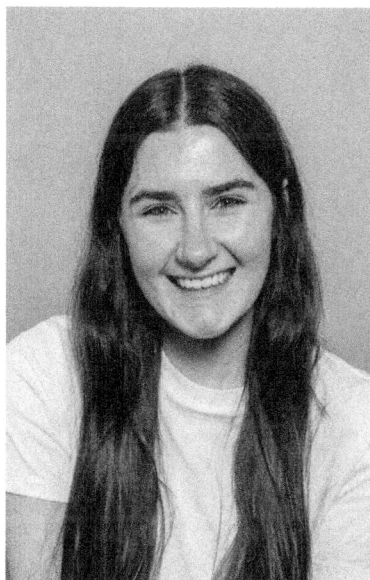

*ZARA BETH* is a content creator, writer and disability advocate based in the UK. She shares content about her life living with chronic illness and documenting her journey with neurodiversity and mental health. She spends most of her time recording videos, reading and writing books, travelling, exploring nature, and can usually be found in bed by 9pm with a cup of tea and her cat.

She has been nominated for National Diversity Awards and shortlisted for a Scope Award for her work in disability advocacy.

# SOCIAL MEDIA

You can find Zara Beth on social media and via her website which can be found using the QR code below.

Here you can also find disability, chronic illness, mental health and LGBTQ+ resources including a Discord Community with online forums, and Zara's videos, music, merch and more.

instagram.com / zara.bethx
youtube.com / @Zara_Beth
tiktok.com / @zeezee25
linkedin.com / in / zarabeth
facebook.com / zara.bethx

Printed in Dunstable, United Kingdom

65374190R00170